Fit to Win

Health, diagnosis
and treatment
in racing pigeons

by Wim Peters

The Racing Pigeon Publishing Co Ltd

Published by The Racing Pigeon Publishing
Co Ltd, 13 Guilford St, London, WC1N 1DX
United Kingdom

ISBN 0-85390-043-4

Text set in 10/11 Century Schoolbook by
RP Typesetters, London.

Edited by Rick Osman.

Cover drawing by Jane Catherall

Cover photograph 'Champion Breakaway' by
Anthony Bolton

Printed and bound in England
by Hillman Printers (Frome) Ltd, Somerset

British Library CIP Data. A catalogue record
for this book is available from the British
Library

Contents

CONTENTS 5

Preface

This book was written from many different aspects.

It all started when friends asked me to examine their ailing pigeons and kindled the interest to delve deeper into the study of pigeon diseases. The desire to prevent the knowledge and experience gained from being lost, was a further prompt towards this publication. The book can be seen as an attempt to bridge the gulf between pigeon racing and science.

It attempts to highlight the conditions that affect the racing performance of apparently healthy birds, including both the erosion diseases and early stages of the fatal diseases. Because a sick bird cannot race, a knowledge of the standard pigeon diseases is essential to an understanding of what interferes with successful racing.

Secondly the book gathers together the current knowledge about disease problems of pigeons, always referring to the effect on racing. Though show pigeons are not specifically catered for, it is true that diseases, acute or chronic, impinge equally on their performances, which necessitate health and form. Knowledge of the disease conditions that can affect pigeons and how to prevent or treat them, is as important to the showman as the racing fancier.

Our knowledge of the diseases of pigeons is still very limited and the book does not pretend to have an answer for every problem. Certain conditions are described for which no explanations are offered but it is hoped that exposure in print will help to stimulate research in these areas. Furthermore, it is hoped that the book may serve as a basis for future improvements; to be updated when new information renders any sections outmoded.

While intended mainly for "lay" persons, it is so that the average fancier has a broad knowledge of and experience in the diseases and conditions associated with his birds and uses medicine on an almost daily basis. Sometimes this leads to unscientific and incorrect use of remedies, resulting in poor results, drug resistance and other complications. Space is devoted to these aspects to prevent their occurence.

No apology is made for facts repeated under different headings if the logical development of conclusions is improved or if the importance of a point is stressed.

Though the book is not strictly scientific, most facts, apart from those indicated, are based upon scientific methods and principles and can serve as reference material.

References have been excluded from the text to make it more readable. They have all been grouped according to their relevant chapters, under Appendix C, Bibliography.

Acknowledgement and thanks is extended to the many fanciers of the Western Cape area in South Africa, particularly Louis, who presented their birds as problem cases and in so doing provided valuable case material.

To my partner, Peter, who, on many occasions, was forced to endure pigeons in the practice and the often untimely attention that was levied on them, my gratitude for your forbearance.

To my dear wife, Herna, who typed the first manuscript and struggled on alone during the many hours that I was preoccupied with this work, my everlasting thanks.

Introduction

Any person desiring success at the game of pigeon racing, must meet three requirements. Without any of these, he is wasting his time, money and efforts, all of which can be not inconsiderable.

The basic requirements for success are:

1. Pigeons of high quality.
2. A logical and systematic management system, meticulously applied.
3. Absolute health of all pigeons in the loft.

In order of importance, I would place the last first. No-one can hope to have success consistently, if at any time the health of his racers is suspect. Top performing pigeons must be super-healthy. (Having said that, it does not mean that sick birds are incapable of recovery, they can and do go on to become winners and super racers.)

Too many times struggling fanciers have culled a season's crop of youngsters, believing them to be inferior, when good health was all they were lacking. It makes no sense to believe that breeding stock, which previously has bred winners and champions, suddenly becomes incapable of breeding offspring that cannot win club races. Nor does it make sense to believe that the other club members have suddenly improved to such an extent that a loft of previously-winning pigeons is no longer able to compete successfully.

It happens frequently that a losing fancier turns to a winning loft, usually in another area and pays dearly for new stock, which are not superior to his own but simply originated from a loft where the management is impeccable and the health is superb.

Many times have we seen losing fanciers become winning fanciers when their pigeons' health was improved. Even top-drawer fanciers occasionally observe their lofts' performances slip but persistently believe that a turnaround in form is just around the corner. They

fail to recognise the subclinical symptoms of poor health responsible for their bad run and, wary of modern medicines, do nothing. If
the reading of this book stimulates such fanciers into taking the
necessary steps, much will already have been achieved.

I have always believed that the sport of pigeon racing should be a
fair contest between fanciers, with the test of skills in breeding the
better racing team, followed by the trial to determine the best
trainer. I would prefer to see all birds equally healthy all the time.
Where's the trial of skills if an adversary has a team of pigeons
which is riddled with worms, while your own is in good health? My
money would always ride on the healthy team of average quality
were they to compete against a sickly team of champions. Let there
be no mistake; a pigeon is sick if it has worms ... or cocciciosis ... or
canker ...etc.

It is said that the 'good old days' of racing pigeons on good food and
clean water are over. Flippant remarks claim that we are now in
the age of clean food and good water and that statement holds some
truth. Some fanciers have been known to want eight days in the
week, to enable them to give all the medications that they believe
their birds need. There certainly is a place for routine controlled
medication but there is probably more danger in the reckless
administration of medications, at dosages that are excessive and
dosages that are too low.

Medicines cannot make a pigeon fly faster. They can only help to
fulfill the bird's potential by eradicating or lessening the effect of
form- and health-destroying diseases. To numerous requests for a
magic, winning medicinal formula there is but a single reply:
Examine the birds to determine whatever it is that prevents their
winning. Treat them, if necessary and if they are good enough,
trained and managed well, they will win. However, no medicine can
make them win.

In previous times, the modern practice of treating for disease, was
frowned upon. Before treatment became more popular, birds in the
most hygienic environment and with the strongest natural resistance, remained healthiest and were the best racers. Now that
medication is aiding pigeons with less natural resistance, speedier
birds often end in front, though they might naturally possess a
lower resistance to disease and would possibly not have been able
to compete successfully 50 years ago. Compare the donkey and the
horse. The donkey's natural resistance to disease is far superior to

that of the horse and it can outlive its more favoured cousin under the harshest conditons – yet not one of us would bet a penny on the outcome if it came to racing.

Together with more refined racehorse breeding, comes a decreased resistance to disease and more dependence on management and medicine to keep health at a peak. Breeding thoroughbreds thus becomes a matter of selection for more and more speed; health becomes a function of hygiene and management – and rightfully so. Our feathered racers are no different.

Most medications are deleterious in some way to the patient, albeit minimally and the most successful way of keeping pigeons healthy, lies in strict hygiene coupled to routine vaccinations and minimal treatment. Strict hygiene however, is difficult to maintain if over-population is allowed to occur. Correct population densities vary with changing weather conditions and ventilation levels, however, no loft should have in excess of two pigeons per cubic metre. It does not depend on the number of free perches, though they also must be considered. To prevent fighting cocks and other forms of stress, there must be "lebensraum", which includes an excess of available perches.

The reasons for culling are varied. Some fanciers believe, correctly, that any bird removed from the loft increases the performance of the remainder, so crucial is population density. In days gone by, sick birds were culled to prevent the spread of disease and because there was a firm belief that sick birds once recovered, were useless as racers. Another function, that of determining the cause of a disease has now been added to the reasons for culling.

Some aspects of a recovered bird merit discussion. The increased knowledge about diseases is so great and the improved diagnostic technology and wider range of available pharmaceuticals so effective, that recovered birds can become good racers, particularly if the illnesses occurred after the birds had fully developed. If permanent injury occurs it results in defective physiological systems, which are reflected in the birds' outward appearance. Any specimens failing to match a physical standard, automatically become candidates for culling.

Pigeons that suffer a permanent physical handicap through disease, have reduced racing futures but provided that a transmissable carrier status does not result (eg. paratyphoid), their breeding capabilities are unimpaired.

Very little is known about the lesser ailments afflicting our birds and much of this is true because most fanciers are quick to put down their sick pigeons. Fortunately today the trend is slowly being reversed and more fanciers are making special efforts to have their birds' illnesses identified. These new investigations are adding daily to our store of knowledge, although conversely they also illustrate very clearly how much we do not yet know.

For example, the controversy rages on over the presence of yellow/white spots in the back of the throat. First trichomonas was blamed, then herpesvirus and E. coli were named and now the spots are believed to be concrements within the salivary glands. Their exact etiology and the significance of their presence, evades us.

What is the role played by the mycoplasmas discovered in the throats of pigeons? They have been discovered and named, but what if any, is their significance in disease and equally important, what role do they play in the race performances of pigeons? Do they cause disease or do they not?

As we proceed, these and other questions will be looked at and possible answers discussed.

• HEALTH IN GENERAL •

Chapter 1

Treatment programmes

Many roads lead to Rome and it is not possible to formulate one system of treatment and management that will be suitable for all styles of pigeon keeping and for every country.

Some fanciers keep their pigeons prisoner during the moulting season, some will let them out for a bath and a fly-around once a week and there are those whose pigeons are out all day to rest, forage or fly as much or as little, as they wish.

So be it. What works for one is not necessarily effective for another. We will sketch principles and broad outlines, to be fitted within the framework of each fancier's own special set of circumstances.

There are three main activities in the calendar of a loft of racing pigeons; moulting, racing and breeding. These seasons tend to overlap each other, some birds are bred from, others race and there are those that do both. Again every fancier acts according to what suits his circumstances.

1. The Moulting Season

The racing season is over.

Preparations for next season begin immediately – if not in physical activity then definitely in mental preparation and planning. Many different methods of management are successful provided that their sole intention is to prepare for next year's racing and the sooner those preparations are begun, the better will be the results and the least problems will be encountered next year.

The single motive behind all activities for the next three months is to prepare the birds for an uneventful moult.

Having just come through the racing season during the course of which they were regularly treated for coccidiosis and crop canker, these treatments are now discontinued. We allow the birds to generate a subclinical level of infection of these diseases to stimulate their immune responses.

Ectoparasite control, that was purposely kept to a minimum, is now strictly enforced.

During the racing season we are opposed to the use of insecticides because of the possibility of poisoning the birds, albeit at a very low level. Nothing must detract from the pigeons' chances of attaining super health, but now the situation is not so critical. Lice and mites are treated for by dipping, dusting or spraying. The chapter on insecticides provides more information.

The loft is cleaned and washed (or vacuumed). Once dry it is sprayed or painted with disinfectant. Every square centimetre of interior surface in the loft must be done, including unused nest boxes and the ceiling.

Our prime objective is to ensure a clean and uneventful moult. We believe in as little disturbance as possible. A setback at this time will not necessarily spell total failure for the ensuing season but negative experiences now, tend to be reflected in negative results during the races. We have seen birds with bad fretmarks, as a result of disease during the moult, go on to have a successful racing season. This is the exception, as poor feathering hampers the ensuing season's racing efforts.

2. The Racing Season

The birds are well-prepared, having been 100 to 150 km along the line of flight in training and are ready for the stressful months that lie ahead. Multivitamin supplementation is increased to twice per week. Because of the erosive quality of coccidiosis and its insidious nature this disease is tested for every month.

Once the season is well under way some opinion can already be formed of the loft's progress. If the management has been good, the treatments regularly executed and the pigeons of a high quality, the results should be satisfactory.

If results are not up to expectations DO NOT RUSH HEAD-LONG TO THE MEDICINE CUPBOARD. A deliberate plan of action will achieve the best and quickest results.

Firstly a systematic and detailed self-examination enquiring into the loft management and re-checking all the routine treatments, must be done.

Ask yourself:

- Were the birds given the best of everything during the off-season?
- Have the birds been given enough time to develop their fitness? In other words was training started too late and was it sufficient? Were the birds entered in races before they were ready?
- Perhaps the start of training was correct but are they now being exercised too much (see the chapter on blue flesh) or too little?
- Are they fed too much or too little?
- Has the food been stored in a dry place away from poisons, rats and mice?
- Is the loft too cold? Too draughty? Too closed-up?
- Are there too many pigeons in the loft? Two per cubic metre is the maximum limit and there can never be too few!
- Were all the routine treatments given? At the correct dose? It is more likely that underdosing has occurred and that though the birds were given the correct medicine, the dose was so low that they were not adequately treated.

Pigeons that appear to be shining examples of fitness and health are not necessarily ready for the rigours of racing. Like all athletes their muscles must be carefully toned for the job ahead. The less overweight during the off-season, the quicker the adjustment to racing fitness. But they can be severely stressed by being brought on too quickly and their progress to top fitness badly hampered by injudicious races early on.

In spite of all treatments being correctly administered, there is no guarantee that they were effective in combating whatever they were intended against. Many reasons exist for such a development; drug resistance developing in the organisms, incorrect medicine dose intake (though correctly administered) through adverse weather conditions with dramatic reduction in water intake, fresh introduction of disease organisms following contact in racing panniers, training or strays etc.

Critical self-examination questions whether every avenue of management was executed with precision and the birds were brought on carefully and slowly, training having started well in advance of the first race.

If we find that the birds are circling well, not flying with open beaks, (an obvious indication that things are not as they should be), but the results are still dismal, we continue the investigation.

The second part of the plan consists of an examination of the pigeons – by a competent person in whom the fancier has absolute trust. The examiner is going to recommend certain steps, possibly

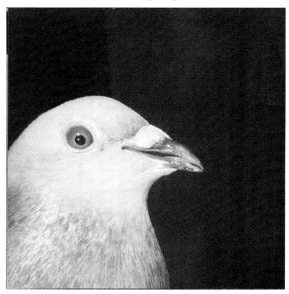

Open-mouth breathing. Many causes are possible so detailed examination will reveal the true reason.

treatment and if there is any doubt about the trust placed in him by the fancier, it is unlikely that his suggestions are going to be carried out. This results in a waste of time and money and in the process the fancier is no further with his problem. (The examiner's view should be an objective evaluation and he will not be swayed by what he perceives the fancier wishing to hear.)

Nor should a fancier be discouraged by the thought of spending some money on a thorough investigation. Having invested thousands in equipment and breeding stock it is false thrift to begrudge the small sum that such an investigation will cost. In return the fancier stands to gain much satisfaction and joy ...... not counting any financial return.

The investigation that is to be carried out will likely follow the outline as set out in Chapter 3.

Notes.

1. Comments on the little secrets that each fancier has and whether they help or not do not fall within the scope of this book.

2. Pigeon preparations that do not state their active ingredients on or within the packaging are not considered for comment in this bookand should not be considered for use on your birds.

3. The various natural and synthetic products used by fanciers to produce form and maintain fitness do not fall within the subject matter for discussion in this book provided that they are not toxic or do not otherwise harm the birds. Whether they are potentially beneficial does not fall under discussion. Some examples are: linseed syrup, bitter aloe syrup, alum extract, Liverine tonic, wild garlic extract, onion extract, various teas, various salts (Epsom salt = magnesium sulphate, sodium bicarbonate, sodium acid phosphate, sodium citrate, Glauber's salt = sodium sulphate, potassium citrate, Kruschen salt which is 80% mag. sulphate etc.) various mixtures containing anything from table salt to creosote, iron compounds, iodine compounds, seaweed extract, carrot juice, anis seed juice, garlic etc.

4. The requirements for grit are discussed under the breeding season. Suffice to say that the birds must at all times have two kinds of grit readily available, ie. shell grit and granite grit.

5. There must always be a multimineral supplement in the loft. Though the specific needs of racing pigeons for various micro-elements are difficult to establish and deficiency syndromes are not often seen, it may be assumed that requirements are at least equal to those for poultry and essential for super health.

6. Fresh soil, crushed old masonry bricks and clay bricks made at home from ingredients such as clay, ash, charcoal, table salt, shell-grit, flowers of sulphur, bone meal and iodine are made available to pigeons under various systems of management. We have not yet come across problems as a result of these products being supplied and they are possibly beneficial.

3. The Breeding season

This is possibly the most interesting time of the year for most fanciers. The challenge to bring to bear all one's knowledge about pigeons and see it embodied in the form of a team of stock birds perfectly matched and designed to bring forth many champions, can only be realised if the pairs are housed and managed under perfect conditions. Any deviations from the perfect state diminish the possiblities of realising the dream, which is a team of champion racing pigeons. Deficiencies in breeding cannot be corrected later.

The pigeons are healthy, having moulted, been treated and rested. If any birds are not well they are removed from the loft, isolated, examined, treated and allowed to recuperate fully before being returned and mated.

No access is allowed from the breeding loft to outside aviaries with earth floors as these become infected with worm eggs and coccidiosis. It is our aim to eradicate worms and this is only possible if the floors of the loft and aviaries are of an impervious material. Once this has been achieved, deworming is at most an annual exercise. Coccidiosis is similarly controlled in the stock loft.

Before the pairs are allowed together, the correct additives are made available. It is essential that the birds have two forms of grit.

Shellgrit is needed as source of calcium for eggshells, bone formation and other physiological processes. The eggshell grit is speedily dissolved and the calcium absorbed and assimilated into the metabolism.

Granite chips act as the pigeon's teeth and grind the grains to pulp, which can be digested more easily by the relatively short intestine. Grinding takes place in the gizzard where the small hard pebbles stay for many months until they become too small after which they are passed in the droppings.

Failure to provide shellgrit will result in;

- soft-shelled eggs
- rough-shelled eggs
- lameness and reversible paresis in laying hens
- reduced peristalsis and egg-bound hens
- rickets in the nest babies.

Ten days after mating the first pairs should be on eggs followed by the others in short succession. The last pair should not take longer than fifteen days to start brooding, any empty nests following this period is an indication that there could be a problem. As an aid to tracking down the cause, see Chapter 10, on breeding problems.

Any medicine that needs to be given must preferably be administered once the eggs have been laid and before the chicks begin to hatch. There are a certain number of drugs that produce temporary infertility and it is unwise to jeopardise the first round of eggs.

Eighteen days after the second egg was laid, the first chick should chip out of the shell. If it does not happen we need to investigate the reasons and take the necessary curative actions.

Summary

- multivitamins are given once per week.
- trace elements and minerals are always available.
- two types of grit are always available.

One thing worth remembering is that the chlorine in some tap water lowers the potency of soluble vitamins. If you live in a highly-chlorinated water area use spring water purchased from supermarkets.

Much the same programme is followed in the following month, but for one exception. The babies have been rung and are requiring protein to grow. This is supplied in the feed. Protein-rich seeds have been given to the breeding birds from the time of pairing but is of particular importance once the nestlings attain the age of ten days.

Whatever the feeding practices, the birds need more than a standard breeding mixture. Commercial breeding mixtures are often short of enough protein for rearing babies, and extra peas, beans, soya, cowpeas or other forms of protein, must be added. The optimum procedure is to feed a standard breeding mixture twice per day and additionally to provide ad lib access to legumes via a hopper system.

If a standard mixture is fed and any feed remaining consists of maize it is a clear indication that the birds are not receiving enough protein.

Feeding pairs experience a big demand for multimineral/trace element additives which must be met. Whether it is for the salt content of these mixtures is not certain (most contain a large percentage of NaCl) but a very strong craving develops in the parents. If not supplied the young squabs do not grow well, suffer from loose bowels, stunted growth and poor quality plumage.

Summary

- multivitamins are given once per week.

- minerals and trace elements are available ad lib.
- feeding mixtures contain extra protein.

Specific treatment during the breeding period is totally dependant upon the fluctuating state of health in each loft. No routine treatments are given. The most common disease to be wary of is crop canker but we do not recommend treatment unless clinical symptoms are seen and believe it to be beneficial for the young birds' immune systems to be confronted with a limited number of organisms while they are in a stress-free environment. Some immunity (premunity) will be developed, enabling them to counter more serious outbreaks of the disease should these occur.

Multivitamins are given once per week throughout the breeding period.

Summary.

- multivitamins once per week.
- trichomonas or coccidiosis treatments only in clinical outbreaks.
- deworming only in clinical outbreaks.
- ad lib supply of shell grit.
- ad lib supply of granite grit.
- ad lib supply of mineral and trace element powder.
- regular cleaning – including unused nestboxes.
- ad lib supply of protein feed (legumes).

Chapter 2

Problems encountered

We assume that fanciers have taken the normal preventative measures and that their birds are free of respiratory infections, coccidiosis, worms, trichomonas and external parasites. In spite of these precautions non-specific conditions will at times become apparent in the loft. We will address these on an informal basis and where the cause of disease is obscure we will discuss possible cause, effect and treatment.

1. Respiratory problems

To be able to deal rationally with problems associated with the respiratory apparatus an understanding of the normal anatomy and mechanics of the system is essential. We will briefly examine the normal and try to correlate the signs and symptoms of the abnormal with this understanding.

The respiratory system

The basic function of any respiratory system is to take fresh air into the lungs so that oxygen and carbon dioxide can be exchanged and then to remove the 'stale' air. Though the physiological mechanisms are the same there is an enormous anatomical difference between the respiratory systems of pigeons and mammals, nevertheless Man's system can be used as a model to compare with that of the pigeon.

A. Anatomy.

Man has a cul-de-sac system. It is closed internally and consists of a trachea (windpipe), bronchi and bronchioli which divide a number of times to end in closed alveoli deep in the lungs. Provision is made for both thoracic and abdominal breathing, both modes being dependant upon the presence of a vacuum in the thoracic cavity. This is effected by a closed thoracic cavity which is capable of expansion and contraction by means of movable ribs and a muscular diaphragm.

The pigeon's respiratory system is an open one, with the lungs connecting at the anterior end with the bronchi and posteriorly to the airsacs. In the place of alveoli are parabronchi from which exit numerous air capillaries, which lie in close apposition to blood capillaries and form the site of respiratory gaseous exchange. The pigeon consequently is said to have a through-and-through type of system, where the lungs are found midway in the respiratory system and do not form the endpoint of air movement. For practical purposes there is no diaphragm and the ribs are immobile, having fused onto the vertebral column, which is rigid except in the mid-back, (equivalent to the thoraco-lumbar junction in mammals) where it hinges. (Some investigators recognise a vestigial diaphragm, divided into two planes and resembling an airsac wall.)

B. Mechanics.

In man the function of both thoracic and abdominal breathing is to enlarge the thoracic cavity. Because the lungs are encased within the chest cavity and are elastic, they can expand and contract in rhythm with the increase and decrease of the thoracic cavity volume. In this movement air is sucked into and forced out of the system. A break in the system, such as caused by a open wound in the chest which destroys the vacuum, makes respiration very difficult or impossible.

The pigeon's lung works like a bellows. Bird respiration is very complicated and has not been fully understood. We will attempt a simple explanation.

The bird's musculature raises and lowers the sternum (breastbone) and backbone, which is hinged between the thoracic and abdominal sections. To inhale the pigeon raises the back and lowers the sternum, causing air to be sucked in via the trachea, through the lungs and down into the airsacs, which act mainly as holding tanks for the inspired air. On expiration the pigeon contracts the abdominal muscles which raises the sternum and pulls down the spine. This decreases the abdominal space, expelling air from the airsacs, through the lungs (where oxygenation takes place) and out via the trachea. The airsacs have a poor blood supply and do not materially assist with oxygen/carbon dioxide exchange.

The mechanism is clearly seen when a sick bird (with respiratory embarassment) is closely observed. To overcome the respiratory deficiency all the actions are visibly exaggerated. It can now be appreciated why a pigeon that is held too tightly, struggles to be free. Breathing is prevented when no allowance is made for the movement of the back and sternum. Suffocation is possible by purely clasping the back and sternum firmly between thumb and fingers of one hand.

Any condition that interferes with free movement of the back and/or sternum causes distress. A hen on the point of lay sits with an egg in the abdomen, which interferes with the movement of her sternum and reduces the volume of air she can pass through her lungs. To compensate, exaggerated respiratory movements are made. If forced to exercise at this stage she would not be able to compensate sufficiently and would cease flying after a while. On a training flight she has reduced stamina, is unable to stay with the pack and arrives home some time after her loftmates.

Though very efficient, being able to function well in a rarefied atmosphere such as found at heights so great that they would incapacitate mammals, the pigeon's respiratory system has distinct disadvantages. Because of the interleading connections between the lungs, airsacs and some hollow bones any infection which enters the respiratory system is readily transmitted to various parts of the body. Secondly, because the airsacs have a poor blood supply they have little resistance to infections. Though the body's primary defence i.e. the antibodies and white blood cells, are present in the bloodstream, they cannot reach the invaders in large enough numbers. Medications are equally affected, in that they fail to reach the site of infection in sufficient concentration, even though they were administered at the correct dosages.

Though the airsacs are separate from one another, their walls are extremely thin and fragile and in practice we find that infective germs penetrate the membrane fairly easily, leading to rapid dissemination of infection. Once an aerocystitis (airsac infection) occurs, there is further mechanical interference with respiration because, having lost their elasticity, the airsacs are no longer able to hold the required quantities of air. The openings with the lungs are occluded (blocked) with pus, infective material and other debris which serve to further reduce free air movement.

On autopsy, severely affected airsacs are frequently seen in conjunction with lungs that are normal in appearance. The lungs have a very good blood supply.

It is not always easy to differentiate a respiratory problem from some other condition in the loft, but careful observation for the following signs will help to recognise the early symptoms.

1.1. WET EYE

Often a wet eye, will be the first sign that something is amiss. It may appear initially as a slight wateriness, possibly with mild swelling of the eyelids particularly the nictitating membrane (third eyelid). This may progress to severe opthalmitis and conjunctivitis with the pigeon rubbing its eye on the wing and causing a wet patch on the shoulder. A wet eye can have several causes and one must attempt to distinguish them in order to assess the future implications.

1.1.1. Most straightforward is an eye or eyelid that is injured when cocks are fighting. No treatment is needed and the injury will heal in a few days.

1.1.2. An early pox lesion developing on an eyelid is can be indistinguishable from a fighting injury or acute conjunctivitis. Examination of the other birds in the loft will indicate whether or not pox is present in the flock.

1.1.3. One-eye-cold as an entity is well-known. It may be the first sign of ornithosis or the result of inadequate or incorrect loft ventilation. If it is a harmless inflammatory condition it will respond to 24 hours of isolation in a pigeon basket, kept warm and out of draughts. If no response occurs the situation is more serious and could possibly be ornithosis.

1.1.4. A sore eye that responds to treatment but is succeeded by different pigeons also exhibiting excessive moisture, at odd times, must alert one to the possibility of ornithosis.

1.2. WET OR DIRTY WATTLES

This may be seen before or even without a sign of a wet eye, but can be definite indication of an upper respiratory problem.

1.2.1. A bit of straw, or other object having found its way into the nostril, will give rise to a wet nose and dirty wattle. Careful examination will indicate if this is the case. Removal of the foreign object results in spontaneous improvement.

1.2.2. Young hens when mating for the first time are inclined to be over-exuberant in their petting activities and sometimes are seen with wattles that are coloured dirty brown, though more dry than wet. Distressing to an inexperienced fancier, the condition is harmless and disappears as soon as the young couple go down on eggs.

1.2.3. A greasy appearance of the wattle progressing to a dirty brown colour, particularly if heard in conjunction with a snick when the birds are at rest (at night), is a sure indication of respiratory inflammation. Often the small forehead feathers just above the wattles are wet and clumped together. Pressure on the wattles produces a dirty brown exudate from the nostrils. Maybe ornithosis is present and immediate action is required.

Wet eyes and dirty wattles in a flock must be regarded as serious and individual treatment is not recommended. If the ventilation and sanitary conditions are good, the affected pigeons may recover after a week or ten days only for new cases to appear from time to time. This may continue for months. A bird that persists with signs or one that clears up only to break down again a few weeks later must be eliminated. It is probably a carrier, resistant to treatment and likely to infect the other birds continuously. These early symptoms may progress to more severe effects of the disease and prolonged treatment must be initiated. See page — for an in-depth study of ornithosis.

1.3. MOVEMENT OF THE KEEL AND BACK

Movement of the keel becomes exaggerated when the bird suffers respiratory distress. This is seen clearly if the pigeon is forced to exercise. After being chased from perch to perch for a few minutes, the bird raises its back and lowers the sternum with each respiration. It sits hunched, low on its legs and appears disinterested on its surroundings. If the condition is severe, open-mouth breathing will be seen. The wings tend to droop and are not held tightly against the body.

It is important to note that, depending on the cause of the condition, the eyes and wattles may be clean and dry. The symptoms are usually observed if there are mechanical problems with the respiratory apparatus, eg. egg-binding, abscessed oviduct, growths of the kidneys, ovary, testes, liver or intestine, abcesses in the adominal cavity, enlarged liver due to cancer, inflammation or mycotoxicosis, ascites, airsacculitis especially if caused by Aspergillus, excessive abdominal fat etc.

Interference with respiration occurs through;

- Interference with the expansion and contraction of the abdominal cavity.

- Occupation of the available space within the abdominal cavity – restricting air intake into the airsacs and through the lungs.

1.4. ROUNDED EPIGLOTTIS

Upon opening the beak, the epiglottis (anterior opening of the trachea) should be a slit-like opening of the trachea, resting loosely on the floor of the pharynx. In the distressed pigeon the epiglottid opening varies tremendously, the worst being an almost round ring with swollen edges. Alternatively it may open and close constantly. This is a sign of severe respiratory distress. The eyes and nose usually are clean and dry.

1.4.1. There are natural and harmless causes for the above condition, these being non-disease impediments to an otherwise well-functioning respiratory system. Most commonly this is seen in overweight pigeons and hens on the point of laying. In these instances the respiratory movements are impeded, particularly in fat birds and the available abdominal air space is drastically reduced. Because it is physiologically normal despite obvious respiratory distress the fat pigeon needs only a corrective diet and excercise, and the eggy hen will be fine a day or so after her egg has been laid.

Some fanciers base their evaluation and selection of breeding stock on the state of the epiglottis. Louis Vermeyen, world-famous pigeon fancier and selector, used this phenomenon amongst other as an important indicator of the racing worth of a pigeon he was asked to judge. He himself did not keep any bird with an epiglottis wider than a slit.

I do not decry this practice but a little caution must be used. It would appear that in some pigeons the epiglottis is naturally very narrow. Conversely we have seen individual birds and certain families of birds, where the opening is more oval. To condemn these birds outright would be a serious error. The facts must be considered against a knowledge of the rest of the family and the conditions. Keep in mind that most breeding birds are unfit and too fat and many amongst these will have oval to round tracheal openings – especially hens.

1.4.2. Pathological conditions causing a rounded epiglottis are numerous and include many varied conditions:

Space-occupying lesions.

All the space-occupying conditions of the abdomen such as tumours, abscesses, oviduct swellings, enlarged organs, etc. can be reflected in visible epiglottid distress. It will be noted that these are basically the same conditions as those responsible for exaggerated respiratory movements. The big advantage of the throat examination is however, that the rounded epiglottis is seen at a much earlier stage – when preventive measures are more likely to be successful.

Fever.

Any febrile condition can be responsible for a rounded epiglottis. The birds may not appear to be ill, but their performances are below normal. Examination of the throat reveals a darker than normal, slightly blueish colour to the membranes of the mouth and throat and a rounded epiglottis, often with swollen edges. The condition corrects itself, usually within weeks, but in the meantime the pigeons are treated by their owner with all the remedies on the market, known and unknown! The etiology is presumed to be viral but as the average pigeon readily develops immunity, it overcomes the condition naturally. Vitamin supplements added to the drinking water is adequate treatment. Excessive stress, such as a very severe racing or training, will tend to prolong and aggravate the problem.

Airsacculitis.

Inflammation of the airsacs has a double effect: fever and toxaemia are present and additionally there is mechanical interference with breathing. Airsacculitis is usually a secondary condition, occuring mainly as result of a neglected primary respiratory disease such as ornithosis. The airsacs are invaded by bacteria, usually E. coli, or fungi, causing inflammation with pus formation and loss of elasticity. This is a severe disorder and I do not believe that these birds will ever again race with success. Treatment for the condition is difficult and usually unsuccessful.

Obstructions.

Obstructions to the airflow will leave the pigeons gasping for breath, with a wide-open rounded epiglottis. It may occur as a result of gapeworm (Syngamus tracheae) infection, which I have never seen in racing pigeons, or more usually, from a plug of inspissated pus, blocking the trachea following bacterial tracheitis. A semi-blocked windpipe cause the bird to produce rales (abnormal respiratory sounds).

Fumigation.

A chemical fumigant causing irritation to the respiratory system mucosa produces inflammation and acute symptoms of distress. Ammonia fumes, formed by droppings that are allowed to accumulate and remain moist, are a common cause in feral birds. These are serious in that they predispose the bird to secondary opportunists, particularly Aspergillus. Less severely affected birds have a good chance of recovery if the hygiene is improved, fresh air is supplied and treatment with antibiotics and vitamins is instituted.

1.5. OPEN BEAK BREATHING.

This is one of the very earliest indications for the detection of respiratory problems.

1.5.1. When held lightly in the hand the beak of a pigeon at rest should be shut. Many pigeons appear to have the beak closed, but careful examination reveals that the beak is slightly open – by about one millimetre. This is not good enough. The upper and lower beaks must lie 100% against each other. Failure of the pigeon to accomplish this indicates that the bird is not ready for racing. It does not necessarily mean that the pigeon is sick and all the facts must be considered before the nearest antibiotic bottle is grabbed for. The ambient temperature could be excessive, the pigeon could be too fat or unfit or could have a mild case of trichomoniasis or mycoplasmosis. Whatever the cause, it must be investigated and corrected, if possible.

1.5.2. Pigeons that appear healthy may be tested for respiratory problems in the following fashion. Hold the beak of the bird closed for a about 30 seconds so that it cannot breathe. Following release the pigeon's respiration should return to normal within a few seconds. Pigeons that are not right, will continue to breathe with an open mouth for a few minutes. They require further investigation.

1.5.3. Hot weather is particularly stressful to birds and Kendeigh showed that the respiration rate in the house sparrow rises rapidly when the ambient temperature increases above 32 degrees C. Calder & King showed that this was true also for the zebra finch and the white-crowned sparrow. From our observations the same seems to apply to pigeons but it is particularly at exercise that difficulties are experienced. The principal methods that pigeons have of shedding excessive heat is to increase their respiration and air all available skin and mucous membrane, thereby increasing evaporation and radiation.

Open beaks often occur in very hot weather especially if the birds are not yet fit. This is regularly experienced at the start of the racing season, particularly if the pigeons were fed too generously. It becomes a problem to get the birds exercising vigorously and the fancier would do well not to overfeed in the off-season, rather rationing the food given to his flock during this period.

1.5.4. All birds with severely embarassed respiratory systems, will breathe with an open mouth, particularly when forced to exercise. Basically the conditions are the same as already recorded in birds showing excessive excessive respiratory movements. See page —

1.5.5. Birds with wet eyes and/or dirty wattles, as described on page 16, will sometimes have an open beak, particularly when held in the hand. These pigeons are highly suspect for ornithosis, with a strong possibility of being carriers of the disease.

1.6. RALES (GURGLING BREATHING)

1.6.1. On occasion rales are heard when squeakers are held in the hand. The young pigeons appear healthy, eat well and have clear eyes and wattles. The parents appear healthy and do not exhibit rales. The signs begin when the babies are already feathered but still in the nest and occur mostly in the hot summer months.

I believe it results as follows; A great deal of water is fed by the parents, some of which spills into the trachea, setting up a foreign body tracheitis with mucus production. Expired air bubbling through the mucus, produces the typical gurgling sound. The problem tends to recur in subsequent nests of the same parents, probably caused by the parental habit of over-exuberant water feeding, particularly by the cock, rather than by an infections agent passed on by the parents.

It is not necessary to treat these babies as the majority will clear up spontaneously within a few days of being weaned and allowed to fly out. Laboratory tests have failed to culture pathogens from such cases. For the 1% or 2% that do not clear up spontaneously, antibiotic injections of penicillin and streptomycin have been very effective. I have known "gurglers" clear up and become champion racing birds, with or without treatment. Others have become great stock birds. There is no justification in culling them, although many fanciers will not tolerate "gurglers" and destroy them forthwith.

To prevent their presence, breeding can be restricted to the cooler months of the year when the cock is unlikely to 'pump' so much water or to cease breeding from the pair, in particular from the cock.

1.6.2. Occasionally rales are heard in an adult pigeon. The bird may not appear to be sick but this is a serious condition and treatment must be attempted.

Injections of Lincospectin, penicillin/streptomycin and tetracyclines have all given satisfactory results. Some birds have remained chronic, intermittent 'gurglers" and on autopsy were found to have had localised, encapsulated airsacculitis. These pigeons would never again have raced successfully but they could have been used for breeding.

1.7. STANDING TONGUE.

There is a firm belief amongst some fanciers that when the tongue of the pigeon does not lie quietly on the floor of the mouth, the bird is not well. A pigeon in respiratory distress will move its trachea and tongue upwards, causing it to stand raised above the lower beak, whereas some birds always present a raised tongue when their beaks are opened. Whether the observation has significance in the absence of other signs, is debatable. I doubt it and am more inclined to ascribe it to a nervous disposition and not a sign of unthriftiness or lesser worth. All observations noted and evaluated, however, have value, it being preferable to observe too much than too little.

2. Droppings

Continuous vigilance is required from dedicated fanciers if they are to detect the first indication when something goes wrong, enabling them to take immediate remedial action. Foremost amongst these daily observations is inspection of the pigeons' droppings, from which valuable information can be gained. A logical approach is essential, however, to distinguish the early signs of disease from normal physiological fluctuations. This is not always easy and requires a clear understanding and knowledge of the normal, transient abnormal and abnormal (diseased).

2.1. NORMAL DROPPINGS

The normal pigeon dropping consists of two parts, namely the brownish pasty ingesta and a topping of white pasty urates. In all birds waste products from the kidney and bowel are excreted as one, because the colon and ureters empty into a common cloaca, which acts as a collecting reservoir and from which the dropping is voided. This can be akward, in that it is sometimes difficult to distinguish between a disturbance of the kidney and intestine.

Whatever the pigeons eat, is reflected to a large degree in the droppings. If the birds are eating a high percentage of maple peas, the droppings will mainly be brown, whereas a mixture of black-eye-susan peas and mealies (millet) will result in a yellowish dropping. Pigeons that have been eating much crushed clay brick (as fed by some fanciers), will pass this in a reddish brown paste (eating soil has the same effect) and those that have been grazing and foraging in fields and gardens will pass droppings of all conceivable colours and consistency, depending on what they consumed.

2.1.1. Green droppings.

These are usually a bad sign in any loft but there are exceptions. When the pigeons have had access to and eaten vast quantities of greens such as lettuce, vegetables or carrot tops this will be reflected in the excreta.

A small, dark metallic-green dropping is seen when birds have not been fed for twenty four hours or more and is seen in nearly all pigeons arriving from a race. It is perfectly normal under the circumstances and occurs because the liver continues to produce bile even though no food is being consumed. Having no gall bladder for storage, bile is continuously secreted into the gut and being bright dark green, stains the scanty gut content a similar colour. The dropping is usually loose.

2.1.2. Loose and watery droppings.

This may be a normal physiological phenomenon when the birds have been disturbed and are nervous and upset. It can occur when pigeons have been exercising, excessively handled, basketed for the first time or frightened by any other unusual occurrence. The colour of the droppings usually does not change and the looseness is of little consequence as the appearance of the droppings quickly returns to normal when the disturbance ceases.

The weather can play a significant role in the consistency of the droppings. During a sudden change i.e. from fine to cold and especially rainy weather, the droppings will very often be seen to become more soft and even loose. It happens because the birds have drunk more water than they require during the wet spell and excrete the excess. Without interference, equilibrium is soon re-established and one must be careful not to upset the rhythm of a fit team of birds by the injudicious use of medicines at this time.

2.2. ABNORMAL DROPPINGS

This chapter deals with the changes in the droppings indicative of conditions that do not necessarily constitute a threat to the health of the pigeons but are more inclined to affect their racing success. Obviously the latter can be a forerunner of the former, making their recognition and management all the more important.

2.2.1. Watery droppings.

Excessive water in either the intestinal part of the dropping or in the urinary part, will result in a wet dropping on the floor. When the pigeon has diarrhoea the greenish-brown intestinal portion varies from soft and mushy to liquid and watery. The white urinary portion is largely unchanged and remains of pasty consistency. Nephritis or nephrosis (kidney problems) is recognised when the white paste changes to a plain uncoloured watery splash with a bit of intestinal content. Because the pigeon is unwell and does not eat adequately, the intestinal portion is also affected, smaller than normal and usually green.

Diarrhoea is an early sign of most diseases that affect pigeons. Generally whenever a pigeon is sick, its appetite is reduced and this is immediately reflected in the droppings, which become small, green and soft. Disease conditions associated with fever and toxaemia cause a loose bowel action.

The most important causes of severe diarrhoea in pigeons are those diseases that have their major effect on the bowel. Foremost are the various forms or enteritis of which non-specific bacterial enteritis is the most common. Other main diseases include paratyphoid, coccidiosis, paramyxovirus, adenovirus, ulcerative enteritis of pigeons, ornithosis, trichomoniasis, hexamitiasis, verminosis especially Capillaria and various poisonings. As these diseases are fully dealt with elsewhere in the book, they are not discussed again.

Polyuria (excessive amount of urine) is seen in most kidney diseases. Paramyxovirus (PMV 1) has a special affinity for the kidney and is one of the few diseases that restricts its effects almost entirely to the kidney (and occasionally to the nervous system). Most other diseases with a systemic effect, affect the kidney as part of their overall pathogenicity. We then see polyuria as part of other disease syndromes. For example, the blood system of a bird with an abscess will become poisoned (toxaemic) and will poison the kidneys though they were not primarily involved in the abscess.

Polyuria without any other sign of illness is seen occasionally in nest babies from ten days of age. Because of the larger volume of water in the droppings, the babies 'squirt' their excreta over the nest bowl. In Belgium and the Netherlands they are known as "spuiters". Lack of adequate protein in the diet and deficient mineral supplementation produces polyuria in squeakers. Some cases of polyuria respond well to dimetridazole (Emtryl), which suggests that trichomoniasis or a non-specific anaerobic infection is sometimes involved.

2.2.2. Green-coloured droppings

As noted previously, a lack of food intake will result in green-coloured droppings, though such droppings, whether loose or firm, are at times seen after normal food intake.

Firm green droppings are often indicative of a liver complaint, particularly when the condition is below-normal. They are regularly seen in cases of 'yellow liver disease' which is discussed in detail in chapter 11.

Loose green droppings are invariably seen when enteritis is present but particularly when caused by hairworm (capillaria) infestation. A pigeon with severe capillariasis passes bright dark green droppings which are slimy and tacky. The gluey consistency is typical of the condition and provides an early clue to the eventual diagnosis which is made by microscopical faeces examination.

2.2.3. Foul-smelling excreta.

During the years 1991-92, many birds died or were lost with foul-smelling bright green droppings as main symptom. An adenovirus infection, complicated by an (pathogenic) E. coli, was responsible. The droppings were voluminous, formed or loose but consistently foul-smelling and green in colour. The pigeons rapidly lost condition. Mortality of 25% occurred in some cases.

A flock of pigeons suffering with mild paramyxovirus infection will at times pass watery droppings but if undisturbed, the droppings can be normal in appearance. Individual droppings do not have a distinctive odour but the collective faeces in the loft, has a characteristic rancid smell, so much so that the presence of paramyxovirosis in a loft can be smelled in the absence of typical symptoms. This is particularly noticeable if the droppings are left to accumulate and not cleared daily.

2.2.4. Normal-appearing droppings.

Although many things may be learned from an observation of the droppings, one may not necessarily assume that all is well if the droppings appear to be normal. A pigeon passing 'normal' droppings may have any from a list of problems.

To the disadvantage of fanciers, the message is that: ONE CANNOT RELY ON THE APPEARANCE OF THE DROPPINGS TO DETERMINE THE PRESENCE OR ABSENCE OF DISEASE. The more important ones, which are typical erosion diseases in this form, are described.

Coccidiosis

Although a true enteric infection, many birds passing 'normal' droppings will, upon microscopical examination of the faeces, be found to have coccidiosis. These birds are not clinically ill. Neither are they healthy enough to race successfully, particularly not over the longer distances. Many veterinarians and laboratories are now offering services to examine the faeces.

Worms

Roundworms, hairworms, proventricular worms and tapeworms

may be present despite the 'normal' appearance of a dropping.

The various species of tapeworm differ markedly in size. The most common type may be seen with careful examination of the faeces. Some pigeons pass up to twenty segments per dropping. Segments can be seen in a fresh sample, a minute or two after voidance, when they will move to the surface and attempt to leave the dropping. The segments are mobile, whitish-pink in colour and fairly small, being just visible with the naked eye. Others species are bigger and may pass eggs within a minute or two of being voided, when the white fluid containing thousands of eggs, is seen.

The existence of other worms is diagnosed by finding their eggs in a microscopical faeces examination. Care is taken with the examination for proventricular worms (Tetrameres and Acuaria spp) as these worm eggs are embryonated and do not float in standard concentration fluids. Direct faeces examination is more reliable.

Paratyphoid

A paratyphoid carrier may appear to be normal in all respects but will shed infective bacteria in the faeces and constitute a real threat to the other inmates of the loft. Bacterial culture of the faeces is the only means by which a carrier of the disease can be identified. To be conclusive, this test must be negative on three consecutive test cultures. Droppings to be collected over a period of four to five days and cultured at one time. No treatment has yet been able to clear up all carriers. Elimination of all birds that test positively is recommended.

Paratyphoid is most frequently found in stray birds that return after a long period living rough. The biggest sources of the disease are from rats or mice fouling the feed and water and from pigeons picking on ground on which dogs have fouled or humans urinated.

3. Lack of condition

Maintaining the optimum racing condition in a team of pigeons is one of the greatest challenges that faces the racing fancier and once the art has been mastered there is little to keep him from top honours. It is generally accepted that the optimum condition cannot be achieved until a successful balance between exercise and feeding, has been attained.

We want the birds to be full-bodied but light in the hand, supple of muscle as if pumped with air. We do not want the birds to be full-bodied, heavy and doughy nor weightless with keels like razor blades.

There are a number of conditions which, without exhibiting overt signs of disease, can prevent the birds from attaining the optimum state. It appears that some pigeons have a stronger innate resistance to disease and that the genetic make-up of these birds allows them to achieve super health, the absolute prerequisite for optimum condition, more easily. I believe that these birds were the best performers in the days before treatments were available.

The obstacles preventing winning condition are known as erosion diseases, the more important of which are;

3.1. Mycoplasmosis.

Around the world there is controversy regarding the pathogenic status of mycoplasmosis. There is no doubt that it prevents winning honours in pigeon racing and is therefore a true erosion disease. It is very widespread and I believe that it is present in every untreated pigeon flock. All pigeons must receive a curative treatment before racing begins, bearing in mind that the organism is difficult to eradicate and that prolonged treatment must be given. Tiamulin, Advocin, Lincomycin, Baytril etc. can all be used for treatment where they are licensed and available.

3.2. Coccidiosis.

Pigeons with coccidiosis are heavy in the hand with solid meaty muscles. They appear to be starving and eat greedily and excessively. When given more exercise, their bodies tend to waste in spite of consuming vast quantities of food. The full-bodied, weightless condition is difficult to achieve and the pigeons are more susceptible to other diseases. Coccidiosis can only be diagnosed by microscopical examination of the dropping, during which the oocysts are easily identified.

3.3. Trichomoniasis.

Optimum condition is well-nigh impossible to achieve if a pigeon has crop canker (trichomoniasis). Most untreated pigeons will be found to infected with the protozoa despite a healthy appearance. The parasites are a constant source of stress to the pigeon and being motile they stray from the upper digestive tract to the respiratory system, where they are irritant and predispose to respiratory infections. The pigeon's defense mechanism is continually active and in the process energy is diverted from the form-producing action which is a prerequisite to winning condition.

3.4. Worms.

Pigeons with worms are not able to realise their potential because of the deleterious effect that these parasites have on the birds.

Roundworms cause pathology mainly by irritating the bowel wall and competing with the pigeon for available nutrients.

Hairworms cause irritation as well as secreting an anaemia-producing toxin; Severe infestations cause anaemia. Pigeons with hairworms are particularly prone to coccidiosis, which is resistant to treatment until the capillariasis is controlled.

Acuaria spp (proventricular worms), produce a severe proventriculitis in addition to which they secrete a severe hepatic toxin. Mortalities are high and treatment is difficult. Thankfully they are very rare in pigeons.

Tapeworms compete for the pigeon's nutrients and cause mild enteritis, usually not severe enough to cause diarrhoea. Cases have been recorded of pigeons that have won races while infested with tapeworms, but these have been easier races and the birds have failed to maintain good condition.

3.5. Yellow liver disease. (YLD)

Unexplained, consistent lack of condition in pigeons, in the absence of other disease, is possibly the best indicator that YLD is present in a loft. The birds eat poorly, train badly and fail to gain condition. Hard training is not possible. With careful nurturing some condition is gained but is lost when the pigeons are raced. Losses are higher than normal and the recuperative period following hard races is extended four or five times. A severely affected pigeon never recovers though it appears to be in good health. Failure to recover body muscle mass is the only noticeable sign. The etiology (cause) of YLD is unknown and treatment relies on careful nursing, vitamin supplementation and selective racing. YLD does not appear to be contagious. The condition is more fully discussed in chapter 11.

4. Blue flesh

Throughout the years much has been said and written about the condition called 'blue flesh'. Whether or not one specific cause only is responsible for the syndrome has not yet been established. Besides the certain knowledge that it exists and that pigeons suffering from it fare poorly in races, very little else is known about it.

The condition is recognised when the skin over the pectoral muscles takes on a dark blueish hue – as opposed to the fleshy-pink colour that is desired. The skin is scaly and rough with small flakes, never smooth and shiny. Blue flesh is often seen in conjunction with a rounded epiglottis and a dark bluish-red colour to the mucous membranes of the mouth and throat. This would indicate that the problem is mainly a respiratory one. It occurs more often during the colder months, disappearing spontaneously at the onset of warmer weather.

Many authors are of the opinion that it is caused by a diet too high in proteins. Racing pigeons perform a highly energetic task for many hours and burn up vast amounts of energy. This requires energy-producing carbohydrates, found in cereal grains. Maize (corn) is a good and relatively inexpensive source. Pigeons that are rationed on seeds containing carbohydrates or oils, are in danger of developing 'blue flesh'.

Limited racing can be accomplished on a high-protein diet, but hard racing is not successful.

The general rule is that the amount of exercise (energy produced) must be relative to the percentages of protein and carbohydrate in the ration.

From the above it would appear that the condition is linked to a metabolic disturbance of sorts and treatment is concentrated on improving the metabolism. A variety of medicinal salts, including sodium bicarbonate ($NaHCO_3$), Epsom salts ($MgSO_4$), sodium citrate (NaCit) and Glaubers salts etc. are commonly used. Switching to a low protein diet is a standard recommendation. A diet of pure clipped barley for a few days is very popular.

An intense scrutiny of the training programme is advised. It appears that the birds are often being overtrained. Most 'blue flesh' is seen at the start of the season. Fanciers are keen but the pigeons, most of which have been held captive during much of the moulting season, are unfit and are suddenly trained beyond the capabilities of their fitness level. From resting for months with only a weekly bath, they are asked to begin circling up to one hour twice daily and in quick time taken on their first training tosses. Many of these birds develop 'blue flesh' from overtraining.

The pigeons are stressed and are not given the necessary time to recuperate. Open lofts during the moulting season with the birds flying out daily, would keep the muscles loose and supple and the pigeons better prepared to begin training. This is not possible for many fanciers and they must pay particular attention to the diet, both the ingredients and the quantity being important.

When pigeons are free to roam, blue flesh is seen when they go foraging, suggesting that poisoning also plays a role. Prevention of the habit and provision of multivitamin/mineral mixtures help to clear the problem.

Our recommendations for treatment coincide very much with the above, remembering that every specific case has varying circumstances, requiring different adaption of the management. The standard treatments for the erosion diseases such as mycoplasmosis, trichomoniasis, verminosis and coccidiosis are routinely given. In addition we recommend regular administration of the B-complex vitamins and high doses of vitamin E. which can be given as wheat germ oil on the food or via the water as Viroban.

Chapter 3

Problems
solving

When all is said and done, racing is about what apppears on the bottom line – which states how many races were won and how much was taken home in prize money. Some do it for the glory or the pleasure, but no-one wants to come last; winning......is what racing is all about. And if we don't win a fair share, something must be wrong. To discover what, where and why that might be and to correct it, is the main objective of this chapter.

Fundamentally there are three possible areas for failure. These are;
1. inferior pigeons,
2. poor management, which includes housing, feeding and training,
3. inadequate health.

The first can only be eliminated once the second and third eventualities have been scrutinised and found to be above suspicion. We will deal primarily with the problems of health but because management is so closely linked to health it is inevitable that certain aspects of management will be discussed.

The question of 'form' arises. What is it and how do pigeons achieve it?

We believe that form is simply the state of physical perfection and fitness that allows pigeons to win races. It occurs when housing, feeding and training are all at optimum level and is the pigeon's physical and mental response to these factors at a time of top health. It means that the bird is not taking medicines, although it is not impossible that the peak condition may have been reached as a result of medicines taken previously.

Viewed from a different angle, we find that when high quality pigeons do not win, it is because of a lack of form, which is caused by substandard management or by poor health.

Certain subclinical conditions which prevent pigeons from reaching top form can be cured by medical means, but, if given time and good management the pigeons' own defence systems can usually also overcome them. Our dilemma is that we do not have time and medication is the surer and quicker way to arrive at the same end. But, no medication or drug is totally without side-effects, so we aim to use medicines with care, lest they do more harm than good.

Procedure for examination.

1. Record keeping

Good records are extremely important as invaluable information gained from a preliminary discussion with the fancier. It may be difficult to obtain the required facts as the owner is usually keen to proceed with the examination of the birds. However patience is vital and gradually clues will be uncovered, not always as an aid to solving a particular problem but certainly as regards the general standard of management.

Knowledge of previous medicines administered is vitally important and usually a list of these, indicating dosages, time and interval given, needs to be drawn up. Inadequate drug treatment has a suppressive effect on most conditions and can be totally misleading as to the real state. For example; Sulphamezathine given for coccidiosis on the day preceding an examination will suppress the disease and render an examination negative for oocysts, leading one to assume erroneously that coccidiosis was not the problem. With all the relevant information to hand this type of mistake would not occur.

Pigeon fanciers tend to be impatient concerning the performances of their birds and rarely allow them enough time to recuperate from an ailment and develop top form. Supposing the birds have hairworms; The fancier suspects this, treats accordingly but, because of only a slight improvement in racing performance next Saturday, help is sought. A negative examination for hairworm eggs results in an incorrect conclusion and diagnosis. In this instance more time was needed for the birds to recover from both the worm infestation and the treatment. Another sequel to this hypothetical case is that because the correct diagnosis was missed, the treatment was in all likelyhood not repeated 10 days later and the possibility of recurrence is good.

Enquiry into the nature of the complaint is made cautiously and the unspoken complaint addressed as much as the spoken. Although the ultimate problem is the lack of racing success, this is not always the reason presented. Complaints include; dry feathers, black tongues, flying with open beaks, failing to circle well, blue flesh, poor training on tosses, slime in the throat and so on. Most fanciers would not seek advice if their birds had any of the conditions mentioned above but were nevertheless winning all their races.

Only one good bird is needed to win and a race may be won even if 19 pigeons out of 20 sent, were ailing. The twentieth can be in good form and win the race. It is unwise therefore, to judge a performance on the results of only one bird – better to look critically at the results of the rest, in comparison to the performance of the pigeons of the other competitors.

2. Clinical examination

Pigeons do not give up their secrets easily. There are not many symptoms that can lead to an accurate diagnosis but some essential features simplify examination. To be able to recognise the abnormal we will briefly look at the normal and make relevant remarks as we proceeed.

The healthy pigeon must possess physical and physiological systems that are all in good working order. Whether or not these systems are functioning normally, will be reflected in outward signs. An attempt to list some of these signs will be made but it must be understood that such a list will be by no means be complete. Each fancier will have noticed peculiarities which occur in his birds at the time of top health, particularly if the birds are related. These peculiarities may be in appearance or in behaviour, but can be reliable indicators of health.

2.1. Behaviour.

The behaviour of the birds should convey the impression of vitality and desire to live. Inside the loft they perform, are vibrant with life, keen to mate and nest, cocks full of fight and hens coquettish. Outside, the birds are eager to fly, taking off into the air at the slightest disturbance. They must want their bath and relish their food.

The flight of a pigeon can reveal its state of health. The sound of the wingbeats of a healthy bird are sharp and crisp, suggesting power and purpose. A pigeon that is unwell or exhausted flies like a glider. The wingbeats are soft, limited in their range of movement and the flight is light and delicate.

2.2. General appearance.

Healthy pigeons shine when the moult is completed. Every feather is in place and the birds' plumage is tight and neat. When they have come smoothly through the moult, the feathers have no breaks, white patches or 'flags' on the feather-tips. The moult was not retarded and all but the latebreds are fitted with a new set of feathers.

The droppings of a fit healthy pigeon are pasty brown with a topping of white and in the early morning covered with down which the bird has shed in the night.

2.3. Feathering.

The quality of the bird's feathering usually is a good mirror of its state of health. Ideally the feathering is tight and glossy, particularly around the neck, and scrupulously clean. Soiled tail feathers are an indication that the pigeon is unwell. By virtue of their perch positions, one above the other, the time inevitably comes when a lower pigeon is bombarded by the droppings of one above. If the targeted bird is healthy, the dropping will roll off it's back but this will not happen if it's condition is below standard. Then the urinary part of the excreta causes white streaks, which, if it happens repeatedly, will leave the tail feathers dirty grey, frayed and tattered.

A quick spread of the wings will reveal stops and frets in the main flights. These are the scars of past illnesses or very hard races and occur when the growth of a quill is interrupted for any reason. Usually they are not noticeable until two or three weeks after the causative event.

The feathers must be supple and shiny with 'oil' spots near the tips of the larger flights. Dryness or brittleness of the plumage is unwanted. Excessively broken feathers point to a lack of resilience, resulting from earlier deficiency or disease.

Evidence of external parasites, such as pinpricks in the large flight feathers, mites and feather lice, should be absent.

2.4. Parasites.

Lice are best looked for from underneath, with the spread wing held against the light. The long feather louse (Columbicola columbae) is found in the vane of the primary flights. Though apparently harmless the presence of lice is an indication of the deficient quality of the general management.

Other lice are occasionally seen but their significance is unknown. They are transmitted mainly from poultry and indicate a lack of proper management. They are chiefly found on the feathers covering the rump.

Feather mites (several species). One species, found particularly on the rump and around the neck, is tiny and barely visible to the naked eye. A small rump feather is plucked from the back and examined in good light with a magnifying glass or microscope to reveal its presence. Another is found adjacent to the shaft, on the underside of the main flight feathers and can be seen if the opened wing is examined against the light. The mites have a predilection for white feathers. The distinction is drawn because the 'rump feather mite' responds to a drop of ivermectin solution applied to the skin, whereas the 'flight feather mite' does not.

The damage done by these parasites is debatable but we have witnessed a losing team come into winning form after the mites were treated. Possibly it was because the birds were able to rest following destruction of the parasites.

Red mites (Dermanyssus gallinae) are severe bloodsuckers. However, they do not live on the pigeon, spending the daylight hours hiding in small cracks and crevices in the loft, emerging at night to attack the pigeons. If suspected that red mite is present, the loft must be visited at night with a flashlight when the mites will be seen as small red spots scurrying away from the light. They are severe blood suckers and can kill pigeons by physical exsanguination. Winning form is impossible to achieve.

The pigeon fly (Pseudolynchia canariensis) is felt as a hard little lump moving rapidly in between and under the feathers of the bird and is difficult to catch. It is a very fast flyer and is sometimes only seen as a dark blur, streaking away from the pigeon. The flies are bloodsuckers, sucking the birds' blood, and causing a great deal of discomfort with their painful bites. (They do occasionally bite humans). An uncomfortable pigeon cannot reach top condition. They transmit pseudomalaria, which can only be diagnosed on bloodsmear examination. If a well-built, well-bred pigeon performs below expectations and pigeon flies are present, pseudomalaria must be suspected and a blood examination requested. However they are rarely seen in Europe.

2.5. The Head.

With the pigeon lying quietly in the hand and completely at rest, the beak must be fully closed. The slightest opening between upper and lower beak indicates respiratory distress.

The wattles are chalky-white and dry. Remember though that young hens when first mating may have brownish discoloured wattles, this is normal.

The small feathers above the wattles on the forehead are dry and unstained and must lie smoothly on the face. Standing forehead feathers are an indication of an unhappy bird, seen with temporary changes in the weather or after a stiff training session. If it is constantly present, cold draughts must be excluded and the quantity of food checked.

The eyes are bright, alert and 'dry' i.e. the eyelids must be clean and dry. Wet eyes may be owing to early ornithosis, pox, a peck in the eye, a wet draughty loft or non-specific conjunctivitis often complicated by mycoplasma.

The pigment of the iris of the eye is bright, regardless of colour, lustrous and obviously healthy. Some diseased or injured eyes may lose colour in the iris, which is usually permanently – cause unknown. Once the eye has recovered, unilateral paleness of the iris is not an indicator of disease. In an anaemic pigeon the iris loses colour and lustre but as the iris colour of some pigeons is naturally pale, this phenomenon is not a reliable indicator. The colour of the tongue and oral mucous membrane give a better indication.

2.6. Throat and mouth.

2.6.1. Colour of the tongue and mucous membranes.

Anaemia is not seen often in pigeons. The colour of the mucous membranes varies from slightly paler than normal to very pale pink and almost white. Severe anaemia is seen in cases of spiral stomach worm (Acuaria spiralis) infestation, when it may be the most striking symptom. Other important conditions causing anaemia are malaria, pseudomalaria, severe roundworm infestations and liver disease.

Inflammation of the pharyngeal cavity causes the mucous membranes to appear fiery red. The condition is frequently seen and indicates a serious problem. The first considerations are trichomoniasis, mycoplasmosis and ornithosis. Toxaemia is seen in enteritis and airsacculitis and is characterised by dirty red-brown changes to the membranes of the throat. Slime is usually very much in evidence in these cases and respiratory distress is common.

Blue tongue. Controversy exits in the fancy regarding the blue-black discolouration sometimes seen at the anterior end of the tongue. Most believe it to be a normal pigmentation (to which group we subscibe) but some consider it a sign of bad form. With generalised toxaemic changes in the body, the tongue shows the same changes, becoming a darker dirty red.

2.6.2. Standing tongue.

Frequently considered a sign of ill-health this phenomenon has dubious value as a diagnostic aid. Other signs are better and more reliable indicators of a pigeon's health.

2.6.3. Spots on the curtain.

Quite familiar to most fanciers are the pinhead or smaller creamy-white spots seen on the curtain, anatomically a flap of the soft palate. Throughout the years the popular pigeon press has, in countless articles and discussions, suggested many causes for the lesions.

It had long been thought that they were the end result of a previous crop canker infection if white and a current infection if yellow. It has been suggested by Viaene that these are signs of pigeon herpesvirus (PHV) infection, although the appearance of the spots has not been associated with disease. If PHV is the etiological factor, it would indicate that the virus is much more prevalent in our lofts than suspected at present and that outbreaks, when they occur as they do sporadically, are probably resultant from additional stress factors. Further research is needed before this phenomenon can be adequately understood.

Microscopically they have the appearance of tonsil abscesses, consisting of lymphoid cell accumulations with a vascular reaction. Various stages of cell degeneration is noted in the lymphoid cells.

Antibiotic treatment does not help to clear them, but it would appear as if spontaneous recovery does take place after some months.

Whatever their cause, experience teaches us that the white spots do not interfere with racing. We have seen birds with spots on the palate, a day later they had won Federation races. Many anecdotes exist to confirm this observation.

2.6.4. Gaps in the curtain.

Gaps in the curtain or the absence of spicules from the lower curtain edge are the result of previous crop canker infection. Provided that the pigeon is fully recovered and free of trichomonads it does not interfere with racing.

2.6.5. Slime in the throat.

This is probably the most controversial issue in pigeon racing. 'Slime in the throat' has been blamed for more failures at racing than any other condition. Showing no other obvious signs of ill-health, the birds are presented because they are not racing well and the desperate owner, opening the beaks, sees 'slime'.

Of the four manifestations of 'slime', three are significant, the fourth being manufactured by struggling fanciers.

a) Clear slime is seen in the throat of many pigeons that are not performing well. It would appear that a secondary infection is set up in the throat, following primary generalised stress-producing circumstances, which vary from coccidiosis, to draughts in the loft, insufficient food, overtraining, worms etc. Correction of the primary cause clears the 'slime' without further recall to medication.

b) Bubbly clear mucus seen behind the tongue at the back of the throat, which is red and inflamed, is a sign that there is a localised inflammatory process in the throat area. This is most usually caused by trichomoniasis, sometimes complicated by a secondary bacterial infection, usually E, coli. Crop canker treatment followed by a course of antibiotics will resolve the condition.

c) Milky-white tacky slime is often seen in the area of and emerging from the epiglottis. The edges of the epiglottis are swollen and inflamed. Often the slime forms a thread from the edge of the epiglottis to the roof of the mouth (Healthy Pigeons, by L.Schrag, 1st. edition, contains a good illustration). The slime differs in all respects from that of the two previous syndromes. It originates from the trachea and is brought up into the mouth via the epiglottis.

Mycoplasmosis has been cited as the etiology by Schrag (1985) and we support this view. The condition responds to antibiotic therapy but is tenacious and difficult to eradicate. It is wide-spread and seen in practically 90% of pigeons at autopsy. It is extremely significant and probably the best indication that mycoplasmosis is a problem in the loft. The indidence in squeakers is low.

On autopsy either the upper 20–30% of the trachea has a thin spread of the slime, or it is concentrated and found as a globlule just inside the tracheal opening. Microscopical examination of tracheal tissues has so far failed to show an inflammation or infection, revealing only an increase in the number of mucus glands one would normally expect to find in this area.

Regrettably, few laboratories are equipped to isolate mycoplasmas from pigeons, which differ sufficiently from those in man and other animals to make their isolation a difficult and costly procedure

d) When faced by non-performing pigeons, some fanciers massage the oesophagus of a bird from the crop upwards to the beak and after a some strokes pull open the beak, peer inside the mouth, see clear mucus and triumphantly exclaim that the bird cannot win because it has slime! This slime is normal in that a certain amount of clear exudate is always present in the oesophagus. For a similar reason birds must not be examined immediately after having been fed. At this time the throat may be hyperaemic and contain some mucus. An hour later would be preferable and give a proper perspective.

If the manufactured slime is turbid, it may result from chronic PHV. These birds will not race. No treatment exists but good disinfection and hygiene help to lessen the effects and duration of the condition.

2.6.6. Epiglottis (anterior opening of the trachea).

Examination of the epiglottis is quick, easy and rewarding. Many top fanciers examine the throats and epiglottis of their birds on a daily basis. The normal healthy pigeon has an epiglottis that is narrow and elongated (slit-like), with sharp edges and small 'spicules' along the sides. The more rounded the epiglottis, the more distressed the bird. However, the shape of the healthy epiglottis depends also on the family of pigeons and on the sex.

Generally speaking the male has a better, i.e. narrower, epiglottis than the hen. An eggy hen will show respiratory distress by having a wider tracheal opening – considered temporary and normal. Deviations from the normal are fully dealt with in Chapter 2.

2.7. Palpation.

2.7.1. Abdominal palpation.

Abdominal palpation has no place on a flock basis. A pendulous abdomen can indicate the presence of a variety of ailments but these are chiefly limited to individual birds. If found widespread throughout the loft, it invariably indicates a severe worm infestation especially the spiral stomach worm, Acuaria spiralis. Anaemia is present and faeces examination for worm eggs will confirm the diagnosis.

   In individual pigeons a pendulous abdomen may indicate ascites, tumours, abscesses, egg-yolk peritonitis, excessive abdominal fat, enlarged liver or similar abdominal conditions.

2.7.2. Muscle palpation.

Muscle palpation is a technique which every serious fancier or examiner of pigeons must attempt to master. The technique is not easy to learn and requires a careful touch and much practice. The large pectoral muscles on the breast bone lend themselves to palpation and their condition is a direct reflection of the physical state of the bird.

   The feel of ideally-conditioned muscle has often been described as comparable to the feel of a pumped-up bicycle tyre – full, yet supple, elastic and 'light'. It is usually found in racing-fit pigeons and lack of it does not necessarily mean that the bird is unwell, the degree of fitness playing an important role. Birds that are too thin, too fat, over- or undertrained etc., usually lose the feel of supple muscle, regaining muscle tension when adequate diet and exercise are given.

   A sick pigeon, however, will not have supple muscles – making palpation a valuable tool for the owner, who can follow the daily progress of his birds. Dehydated muscles feel doughy and flat with the skin wrinkled and without elasticity.

   Loss of muscle suppleness in pigeons on an adequate management system, is a flickering warning light to the aware fancier, who should immediately take further steps to determine the source of the deterioration.

3. Five simple tests

A few relatively simple tests can be done to gain better insight into what might be at the source of a problem. A group of birds that is underperforming, is presented for examination. We assume that these birds have had all the necessary routine medications, are being managed satisfactorily and are without disease on clinical examination. Routine examinations are now done for the following conditions.

3.1. Coccidiosis

Coccidiosis is the scourge of successful pigeon racing. Previous treatment is no guarantee that the disease is under control. Pigeons treated as recently as five days before examination have been found to have had more than acceptable numbers of coccidia oocysts in their droppings.

Test as follows : a small dollop of fresh droppings (about one to two grams) is placed on a microscope slide, being careful not to include the white urine deposit in the sample as this will make the examination more difficult. Enough water is added to make a thin emulsion. The faeces is spread thinly and evenly over the slide. If the sample is too thick the oocysts are superimposed on faeces material, which makes their identification more difficult. The examination for the presence of oocysts, which appear as small oval bodies with an eccentral content, is done under intermediate power, 100 X magnification.

The number of oocysts passed is dependant upon the degree of infection, the amount and time interval from the last meal and the time of day. Very rarely no occysts are found. Do a direct examination because it is quicker and because a concentrated sample is almost never free from oocysts, leading to confusion. I find that four or less oocysts per microscopic field, is an acceptable level and treat all pigeons with 5 or more. Taking specimens from about 5% of the birds gives an adequate representative sample of the loft and I act according to the severity of infection of the worst case. The others do not suffer from the treatment and it reduces the spread of the disease.

3.2. Worms

When examining for coccidiosis, as above, simultaneous examination is done for the presence of worm eggs. We believe direct examination to be better and reserve flotation techniques for special situations. The procedure will reveal the presence of roundworms, hairworms, Tetrameres spp, Acuaria spp, flukes and some tapeworms.

A refined flotation technique may be done as follows but the method is not successful for the heavier embryonated eggs of Acuaria and Tetrameres. About 2 grams of faeces is mixed with 5 ml water to make a soupy suspension and to this is added 5 ml of saturated sugar or salt solution. All is well mixed and left to stand for thirty minutes or centrifuged for three minutes.

The eggs float and accumulate at the top of the mixture, where they can be collected by lightly touching a flat surface to the top of the fluid so that a few drops adhere to the carrier. These are transferred to a glass slide and examined. The presence of only one worm egg is sufficient cause to implement a course of treatment.

Certain tapeworm species pass eggs in the droppings whereas others pass ripe segments. The motile segments can be seen with the naked eye as they leave the dropping a few minutes after it has been voided.

3.3. Crop canker

Crop canker organisms are naturally present in most pigeons and I believe that their presence, even in the slightest degree, has a deleterious effect on performance. To test for them is a simple procedure. A long cotton bud is dipped into water and the excessive fluid squeezed out. With the bird's neck stretched, the bud is passed through the mouth, down the oesophagus into the crop and moved gently up and down against the side of the throat and crop. Upon retraction the soaked bud is sqeezed onto a glass slide and the liquid microscopically examined at intermediary power (100 X magnification). It is recommended that 5% of the birds in the loft are tested.

Trichomonads are seen as small pale organisms moving haphazardly in small circles or clumped together in small groups that appear to vibrate. Usually, in untreated pigeons, the field is covered with parasites and treatment is essential. In treated lofts some birds are clear, whereas other birds might have a severe infection. The state of the severest affected pigeon is used as a guide to decide about treatment. If only a few parasites are seen in each member of the test group we recommend treatment, but delayed for one or two weeks.

3.4. Feather Mites.

Although not pathogenic, we believe that the presence of feather mites is a disadvantage. Larger mites are seen on the main flight feathers, particularly if white. For the examination for smaller mites, a body feather is plucked from the rump, just anterior to the tail and examined under low magnification, (40 X enlargement). Mite eggs, nymphs and adult mites may be seen, treatment advice in the racing season depending upon the degree of infestation. During the moulting period we recommend treatment if a few mites are present. It is not unusual to see 10 or more mites per feather.

3.5. Protozoan blood parasites.

A drop of blood is taken from the foot by puncturing the skin with a sharp needle. Best results are obtained if the side of a toe-pad is gently pricked between the skin scales – usually this will provide a small drop of blood, which is all that is required. The toes can bleed profusely, so that care must be exercised when the blood is drawn. A blood film is made on a glass slide, fixed with ethanol and stained with Stevenol Blue (Giemsa or another suitable stain is also acceptable). Examination under the oil lens (1000 X magnification) will reveal the parasites.

Pseudomalaria (Haemoproteus spp).

Though pseudomalaria is not usually apparent as a clinical entity the disease has a detrimental effect on normal physiology and therefore on racing performance. When doing a routine clinical examination this condition is included in the battery of diseases under scrutiny. Diagnosis is made by demonstration of the parasites in the cytoplasm of the red blood cells. Treatment occurs with primequine phosphate or any other effective anti-malarial.

Malaria. (Plasmodium)

Malaria causes a severe clinical disease with anaemia but is very rare indeed. Problems can arise with the differentiation from Haemoproteus on bloodslides but the clinical picture dictates treatment.

4. Autopsy

Having progressed through the history, and done the clinical and microscopical examinations, the source of the problem may still evade the examiner. An autopsy is the final resort and often provides answers that are not obtainable by other means.

The carcase must be fresh. Autolysis begins immediately after death and makes accurate diagnosis very difficult, as colour changes rapidly occur, especially in the liver and intestines.

The autopsies done on other birds (eg. breeding birds) are also discussed here. In this respect the differences in the growing pigeon, between the proportions of organ size to body size, must be recognised. These are wholly adapted to the purpose they perform.

At 3 to 5 days of age the intestine, liver and pancreas comprise approximately 30% of total body mass, as against 10% in the adult bird.

In the young bird the urinary system is large. At 21 days the kidneys are 165% of the adult pigeons's kidneys. The spleen is similarly enlarged.

The Bursa of Fabricius reaches maximum mass at 3 months.

4.1. External features

A thorough external examination is carried out. This reveals whether the carcase is fat, thin, dehydrated, and has obvious lesoins on the face, feet, around the anus or inside the throat. Soiling of the feathers around the vent give clues as to the digestive and urogenital tracts. Slimy mucus is invariably found inside the throat and is to be very carefully evaluated in the light of other findings, as it may be of no significance in a dead bird. Conversely, white mucus originating from the inside of the trachea is significant.

Defeathering the breast, abdomen and neck is done before the autopsy can be performed. Using a magnifying glass or microscope the feathers are examined for mites and lice. With the pigeon lying on its back, the skin between each leg and the body is cut through. The legs are forced upwards and dislocated out of their sockets so that the bird lies spreadeagled.

With scissors an incision is made through the abdominal muscles and ribs to separate the keelbone from the back. The incision is continued on each side up to and through the shoulder bones, taking care not to enter the crop. The whole breastbone with the pectoral muscles can now be lifted off to reveal the internal organs. When lifting the keel, the airsacs are carefully examined before cutting through them to fully free the keel. If the pigeon has been recently killed, cotton wool is kept at hand to soak up the blood which oozes and obscures the view. The skin of the neck is stripped off up to the head. At the beak the skin is severed and discarded. The internal anatomy is now revealed.

Before the detailed autopsy is continued, the internal carcase is examined in general. It is noted whether the carcase is pale and anaemic or dark, dehydrated and toxic, fat or thin, and immediate clues as to chronicity, verminosis, poisoning, etc., are seen.

First impressions are important. The examination is continued, even should the apparent cause of death or disease be discovered. All systems are meticulously examined as more important changes may yet be found.

4.2. Cardiovascular System

A bright cherry red colour of the blood is seen in cyanide poisoning (water in mine dams).

The great vessels at the base of the heart can rupture, causing acute mortality.

Internal gout is recognised when the liver, intestine and heart is covered with a layer of crystals.

In cases of severe mycoplasmosis, compicated by bacteria the pericardial sac may be thickened and opaque from infection and inflammation.

4.3. Digestive system

The inside of the mouth and throat is checked for signs of pox, trichomoniasis, herpesvirus or other lesions. The growths are incised to examine their inner structure. Diphtheric pox forms fleshy growths covered with yellow exudate – whereas the growths seen in canker are yellow caseous throughout. Other birds in the loft are examined for external signs of pox. The mushy exudate of pigeon herpes virus (PHV) is non-adherent.

The oesophagus is sliced open to the crop and the lining examined. Moniliasis of the crop is differentiated from canker. Monilial plaques are white in colour and the underlying crop mucosa is thickened.

The crop content is examined. If the crop is full we know that the bird was not sick for very long. We look for poisonous materials or seeds such as Sesbania. Finding snails or insects, indicates that the pigeon was foraging on open land and suggests the possibility of poisoning or internal parasites.

An empty crop suggests that either, the bird vomited (check history), was not fed or did not eat. A small amount of creamy mushy content with or without food, suggests subclinical PHV in an adult bird.

Smelling the crop and crop content can give an indication of moniliasis, poisoning, PHV (foul smell) etc.

The crop wall is thickened in rearing (normal), moniliasis and trichomoniasis (microscopic test).

The oesophagus at the thoracic inlet between the crop and proventriculus is a favourite and lethal site of trichomoniasis. In the confined space, an inspissated abscess, causes obstruction of the oesophagus and trachea, leading to starvation and severe respiratory distress. The canker 'growth' penetrates the oesophageal wall and is invasive in the surrounding tissues.

The proventriculus is the favourite location of the parasitic worms, Tetrameres and Acuaria. The females of Tetrameres invade the proventricular wall causing damage to the glandular structures. The worms are seen as red blotches of match head side both from the outside and inside of the organ. Pressure on the stomach wall will cause them to pop out into the lumen of the stomach. A scraping of the interior lining of the proventriculus, examined under the microscope reveals the presence of the thin threadlike male worms of Tetrameres. Marked thickening of the proventricular wall occurs.

Adult Acuaria spiralis attaches themselves onto the inside of the proventriculus and by burrowing with their heads into the wall, excite an intense inflammatory reaction. There is severe oedema and proliferation of the mucosa with the formation of slime "bubbles". The reaction is so severe that the causative parasites are hidden under the inflamed tissues, which must be cleared away before they become visible, firmly attached to the proventricular wall. Marked thickening of the proventricular wall occurs.

Focal haemorrhages are seen in the proventriculus with Sesbania seed poisoning and in Newcastle disease.

The gizzard does not undergo much change in disease. The thick lining is normally stained a yellowish-green colour. If the bird has been sick, or was not fed for a few days, the lining is stained bright metallic green. A pigeon returning from an overnight race could demonstrate this and care must be taken not to attach too much importance to this change. If the bird has been dead some hours, the horny layer strips easily from the organ. In insecticidal poisoning the horny layer, usually firmly attached, comes away easily.

Localised necrosis of the horny layer has been seen in cases of vitamin B12 deficiency. When no other pathology is found the etiology and significance of the change is unknown.
Foreign bodies such as nails or bits of wire, swallowed by hens in particular do not pass through the gizzard and often the forceful contractions cause it to penetrate the wall of the organ. Depending on the direction of penetration, various conditions may result such as muscle abscess, peritonitis, liver abscess etc. The result usually is fatal and on autopsy the bird is emaciated with the obvious foreign body damage.
The intestine must be extricated from its normally coiled position and laid out on the examination table in linear fashion. In pigeons the caeca are very small and insignificant. For our purposes no distinction will be made between the large and small intestine.
External changes to the bowel are first noted. Roundworms cause enlargement and thickening of the intestinal wall, which assumes a turgid character in place of the normal softwalled appearance. The colour is paler than normal. In acute haemorrhagic enteritis the intestine becomes thinwalled, red, inflamed and flacid and contains more fluid than normal. The fluid may be bloodstained.
The ulcers seen in ulcerative enteritis of pigeons, paratyphoid and non-specific enteritis, appear as discreet raised areas on the serosal surface. Debris from such ulcers can occlude the intestine with typical ballooning with liquid ingesta, semi-solid in parts, anterior to the lesion.
The length of the intestinal tract is sliced open and examined. The duodenal part of the gut is usually slightly more red and thicker than the rest of the small intestine (predilection site for coccidiosis).

Roundworms (ascarids) are readily seen but unless looked for microscopically hairworms (capillaria) can be missed. A light mucosal scraping to collect intestinal material is examined under low power to reveal the presence of the thin hair-like worms. The females are often seen full of eggs. Should a microscope not be available, the hairworms can be seen if the intestinal content is scraped off, squashed between two glass slides and held up against a good light for viewing.
Some tapeworms of the pigeon are extremely thin and threadlike

and easily escape observation. A mild enteritis is caused. Grasping a small amount of intestinal content between the blades of a pair of forceps and lifting it from the bowel, will reveal thin stringy threads. When examined microscopically these are seen to be tapeworms. Washing the intestinal content will also reveal the tapeworms – seen more easily against a black background. Vast numbers of parasites may be present with surprisingly mild pathological changes.

Enteritis appears in many forms. In the peracute form, where the pigeon has died very suddenly (eg. caused by Citrobacter freundi), the gut wall is red and thin and the intestine has a watery or haemorrhagic content. A more chronic form of enteritis, such as seen in coccidiosis, reveals a slightly thickened reddish intestinal mucosa in affected areas, while the rest of the bowel appears normal.

Ulcerative enteritis of pigeons, etiology unknown though probably a virus, occurs less frequently. Discreet ulcers are seen throughout the length of the bowel although certain areas are more affected than others. Ulcers in the bowel are occasionally seen in cases of paratyphoid (salmonellosis) and candida albicans infection. On the mucosal surface the ulcers have a definite raised circumference – resembling a small flattened crater. The colour of the ulcerated area is the same as normal tissue.

E. coli can cause extensive ulcerated areas, with debris from the lesions blocking the intestine, causing accumulation of ingesta anterior to the obstruction. Accumulated green-black semi-fluid causes enlargement of the bowel circumference. The bowel diameter may be three or four times the normal.

The liver is an important organ for regulating the health and racing condition of the pigeon. It is affected by many conditions as part of an overall disease e.g. paratyphoid, PHV, adenovirus, mycotoxicosis, trichomoniasis etc.

Swelling of the liver is seen in paratyphoid, where it often occurs together with patchy pale-greyish necrotic spots of varying size. Larger discreet abscesses in the liver can be caused by trichomoniasis and tuberculosis. A swollen liver diffusely yellowish-pink in colour from fatty degeneration, occurs in chronic ornithosis. Pinpoint haemorrhages in a swollen liver are seen in cases of erysipelas infection.

Other bacterial infections of the liver result in swelling and colour varations from greenish black to purplish black and all shades in between. Clostridia, coliforms and enterococci have been incriminated in bacterial hepatitis. Pseudotuberculosis (Yersinia infection) causes enlargement and pale miliary nodules throughout the substance of the organ.

Severe enlargement of the liver may be caused by tumours of which leucosis is the most common.

Atrophy of the liver is seen in chronic disease conditions where the carcase is cachectic. Severe Acuaria infection causes anaemia and marked liver atrophy.

Pancreatic changes are not often seen. The colour of the normal organ which is light pink, pales to almost white in cases of severe anaemia. The pancreas may be a dark dirty pink when the bird is feverish. In severe cases of herpesvirus infection the pancreas has appeared pale to white.

The spleen is capable of tremendous variation in size and most infectious processes cause a splenomegaly. Ornithosis, herpesvirus and pseudomalaria are the main causes for enlarged spleen and may cause it swell to 5 times the normal size. The enlarged spleen is dark, almost black and markedly enlarged. When this is encountered, a liver impression slide must be examined for ornithosis and a bloodsmear checked to rule out pseudomalaria. Acuaria and Tetrameres cause enlargment of the spleen to a lesser degree.

4.3. Urinary system

The urinary system consists of two multilobed kidneys and ureters which empty into the cloaca. Few changes are seen. Nephrosis occurs in paramyxovirus infection and is often the only pathological change evident. It also occurs as a complicating factor in most other severe disease conditions.

Tumours of the kidney occur occasionally but their relative frequency has not been tabulated and their occurrence is sporadic. Anaemia is reflected in the kidneys by paling of the organs and occurs particularly in Acuaria infestation and malaria. Localised pale areas with swelling is evident in paramyxovirus infection. Bacterial nephritis such as paratyphoid causes localised pale areas. Pseudotuberculosis causes discreet pale swellings in the kidneys as part of a general infection. Swollen pale kidneys are seen in cases of salt poisoning.

Severe swelling of the kidneys to three times the normal size with interstitial nephritis has been seen, frequently accompanied by gout. The ureters are clearly visible, filled with uric acid. The kidneys have a glistening appearance. A virus infection is suspected but the exact etiology remains obscure.

4.4. Respiratory system.

Tracheitis is rarely seen in pigeons. A localized granulomatous tracheitis, of unknown etiology and apparently infectious, is occasionally seen. The lumen of the trachea at the affected area becomes decreased and the bird experiences difficulty in breathing, eventually dying from suffocation and general malaise.

We have not seen gapeworms (Syngamus trachea) in pigeons elsewhere but they have been reported. They are bright red in colour, embedded on the tracheal lining and cause a severe mucohaemorrhagic reaction. Severe infestations may cause mortalities from asphyxiation. The relatively large eggs are coughed up, swallowed and passed in the faeces.

Mycoplasmosis causes a milky-white slime in the trachea in nearly all birds that we examined. At autopsy the slime occurs at or near the epiglottis as a collection of white tacky mucus or it is spread as a thin layer covering the internal mucosa down the length of the trachea. The amount of slime is variable but usually consists of 5 to 10 drops. Histopathology of the trachea reveals an increased number of mucus glands without evidence of an inflammatory reaction.

Pneumonia. Acute purulent pneumonia is caused by Aspergillus fumigatus in young pigeons; No treatment is advised but the management is altered. Aspergillus is normally contracted from straw that has been exposed to moisture.

Chronic encapsulated bacterial abscesses occur in the lung and can become active if the immunity is broken down eg. when steroids are dosed. Chronic aspergillosis can cause plaques of growth in the airsacs, spreading into the lung.

Aerocystitis (inflammation of the airsacs) is not a common problem of pigeons. It usually occurs secondary to a respiratory infection or perforated abdominal disease. The airsacs may be thickened and slightly opaque, or resemble thick whitish/yellow membranes covered with pus. In the latter cases the infection is wide-spread and covers all the abdominal organs and intestines. The causative organism is often E. coli. Pseudomonas aeruginosa has also been incriminated, in which case the disease is very refractive to treatment. Concurrent liver, spleen and kidney pathology is not unusual.

Acute aspergillosis is seen as a primary infection of especially young pigeons. It presents as an acute purulent pneumonia and aerocystitis with bright yellow semi-liquid pus in the affected areas. The condition is rapidly fatal and does not respond to treatment. Chronic aspergillosis of the lung may be confused with the grey/white spots of paratyphoid.

Chronic aspergillosis affects mainly the abdominal airsacs and lungs and usually occurs as a secondary invader. The disease may be seen as small discreet plaques, grey-green and "hairy", distributed throughout the abdomen, to large blotches or ball-like sacs inside which the typical fungal growth is seen. The lungs are seldom affected, but lung absesses occur occasionally and are obvious as large caseous solid areas in the normally spongy lung tissue.

4.4. Musculoskeletal system

The muscles reflect to some extent the pathology within the other systems.

Chronic paratyphoid is seen in the musculature as small grey areas, similar to the abscesses seen in the lungs. The muscles appear wasted and doughy.

The joints are severely affected in some cases of paratyphoid infection, particularly in young birds. The wing butt joints are very susceptible.

Pseudotuberculosis is recognised by miliary creamy nodules, scattered throughout the carcase. Some nodules are seen in the musculature.

Deficiency symptoms of calcium are seen in the skeletal structure, which is underdeveloped, malformed and soft. Bones are easily broken.

• DISEASE CONDITIONS •

Chapter 4

Viral diseases

The virus responsible for causing Newcastle disease in chickens has been isolated from pigeons on a number of occasions but rarely affects pigeons, and only causes outbreaks when special conditions are present. There are few reports in the literature. Agricultural authorities are mainly concerned with the virus in pigeons insofar that it is able to be spread by them, both biologically and mechanically.

In 1981, a new disease was reported in pigeons. It was highly infectious and resembled Newcastle disease of chickens in certain respects. Extensive laboratory tests eventually diagnosed the causative organism as being a variant of paramyxovirus 1, the etiological agent of Newcastle. Because both viruses, the original and the variant, have been described and isolated from pigeons, we will deal with each one separately.

1. Newcastle disease

Etiology.

The causative agent of Newcastle disease (after Newcastle-upon-Tyne where it was discovered in 1926), is a myxovirus in the parainfluenza group. It causes a highly contagious disease of all birds particularly poultry with mortality ranging from 2% to 95%, depending the strain of the virus. The virus is extremely resistant, having survived for 255 days at temperatures ranging from minus 11 degrees C. to 36 degrees C.

Eisa & Omer showed that virus isolated from pigeons was shown to be apparently indistinguishable from chicken isolates.

Symptoms

Palmer & Trainer reported that pigeons primarily developed central nervous system signs, including in-coordination, opistho-tonus, torticollis, paralysis, tremors, and sleepiness. Respiratory distress is seen less frequently, although an increased respiration amd open-mouth breathing occurs. Forehead feathers are soiled and diarrhoea is seen. Transmission takes place mainly via direct contact.

Sudden onset of listlessness, inappetence, nervous manifesta-tions and inability to fly were reported by Eisa & Omer. Crippling, torticollis and partial to complete paralysis persisted in surviving birds.

Pathology

Ullrich & Sodan found that the lesions in pigeons resemble those in fowl. These are seen mainly in the upper respiratory system with hyperaemia, mucus plugs, congestion, haemorrhages in the trachea and exudate in the upper respiratory tract. Tumor splenis and catarrhal enteritis may also be seen. Haemorrhages in the proventriculus are regarded as pathognomonic.

Severe losses (100% morbidity and 80% mortality) were reported from an outbreak in Sudan, but post mortem examination showed hardly any noticeable gross lesions.

Diagnosis

Similarity with other diseases makes the diagnosis of ND on autopsy suspicious and laboratory confirmation is essential. The techniques of virus isolation are difficult and several quick and easy serological tests that rely on the demonstration of antibodies to the virus are used. ND must be differentiated from ornithosis, mycoplasmosis, non-specific encephalitis, paratyphoid, nutritional deficiencies, enteritis, haemorrhages in the proventriculus caused by Sesbania poisoning, mycotoxicosis and sulphaquinoxaline poisoning.

2. Paramyxovirus (PMV)

The correct name would be paramyxovirosis or paramyxovirus infection but in the language of the fancier 'paramyxovirus', shortened to paramyxo, has become so deeply rooted and universally accepted, that it would cause unnecessary confusion to attempt modifications at this stage.

History

The disease was first reported from Egypt and Sudan in 1981. In 1982 it occurred in Belgium following the importation of two pigeons from Italy. During the next two years the disease spread rapidly throughout Europe and to the rest of the world. In South Africa the disease was first suspected in the early summer of 1984. Subsequently outbreaks have been reported elsewhere and the causative virus has been identified and confirmed by comparison with the European etiological agent.

The virus

Serological studies of virus isolates collected from various European centres, showed conclusively that all isolates belonged to type 1, paramyxovirus serotype of avian paramyxoviruses, of which seven have been identified. Avian paramyxovirus 1 (A/PMV 1) is well-known for its ability to cause Newcastle disease in chickens. The pigeon isolates were demonstrated by serological studies to be both similar to and distinct from A/PMV 1. Their binding and haemagglutination inhibition properties with mouse monoclonal antibodies gave belief to the fact that the pigeon virus was a variant of A/PMV 1. Pigeon isolates from different countries, possessed the same serological properties, showing that the virus was identical to the one that caused disease in North Africa.

In 1981 it was shown that the virus isolated from an outbreak of viral encephalomyelitis in Iraq in 1978, presumably caused by pigeon herpesvirus, could be an avian paramyxovirus type 1. In 1985 it was shown that the virus was apparently identical to the variant A/PMV 1.

Symptoms and Course of Disease.

The incubation period varies from one to six weeks, so that many pigeons in the incubation stage and considered healthy, are sent to races and shows, disseminating virus in vast quantities. Virus excretion is highest at the end of the incubation period and shortly after the onset of signs.

The symptoms are grouped into four different categories:

1. The most common and first-noticed sign, is a profusely watery dropping, which results from interstitial nephritis and polydipsia. The normal pigeon dropping is pasty and formed, consisting of a brownish intestinal portion with a topping of white urates. In the diseased bird the intestinal portion becomes green (because the bird is sick) or is absent and the dropping appears as a watery splash with or without a portion of green faeces.

The polyuria may be severe and the loft floor become wet, with a typically rancid, foul odour. Young birds fail to grow properly and loss of condition is apparent. Older birds appear to be healthy, eat quite well, display and breed but fail to gain racing condition. Race results are poor and losses high. Post-race recovery is markedly prolonged.

Excitement aggravates the polyuria. In mildly affected lofts the droppings appear normal and formed in the morning, only to worsen during the course of the day, with many birds passing typical watery excreta by evening. Resistance to other disease such as coccidiosis, trichomoniasis, aspergillosis etc., is be markedly reduced.

2. Dramatic symptoms are seen when the central nervous system is affected and problems with balance predominate. Initially a fine tremor of the head, which may or may not progress, is all that is noticed. More severe symptoms include various degrees of torti-collis (twisting of the neck or stargazing is common), circling, stag-gering, leg or wing lameness, somersaults upon attempting to fly etc. Affected birds peck at food and miss, resulting in loss of condi-tion and starvation. Nervous symptoms become exaggerated when birds are excited. Central nervous systemn disturbances, seen in about 5% of pigeons, occur at the onset of the disease.

Lameness occurs in the wings and legs but in contrast to paraty-phoid, no swellings or other external signs are seen. Lameness may prevent a bird from flying and the affected wing will droop, causing the last primary flights to be soiled as the wing is dragged on the floor.

Mild nervous symptoms usually disappear in a few weeks. If the pigeon manages to eat and stay alive a severely affected bird may yet "recover" even up to one year after first showing signs (take-over function of the brain tissue?). Valuable birds must therefore not be destroyed, but maintained for at least twelve months after

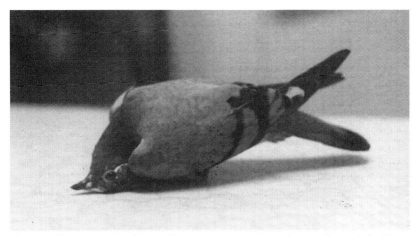

A typical 'stargazer' suffering from paramyxovirus, the condition is indistinguishable from paratyphoid and non-specific meningitus without tests.

the first observation of disease. Affected pigeons can rear normal youngsters.

3. Occasionally young chicks in the nest die suddenly, without showing any previous indication of disease – they are in good condition and have a crop full of food. The occurence is rare, but may be one of the first indications that PMV is present in the loft. Alternatively nestlings become weak, thin, emaciated, dehydrated and die, in which cases it is usually found that one or both parents are also ill. If breeding is continued, mortality in the parent birds will rise. We advise the culling of all youngsters that are not well, followed by the administration of inactivated vaccine to breeding stock and cessation of breeding for six to eight weeks.

4. Feathering problems take many forms.

Formation of a 'flag' at the tip of a feather is typical and only seen with PMV. It may drop off, leaving the feather slightly shorter and with an untidy feather tip.

Feather follicles that are affected result in a malformed, twisted flight or a total lack of feather growth.

PMV in nestlings at the start of feather growth, causes the squab to develop white patches near the ends of its feathers. The discolouration results in a remarkable grizzling of the expected

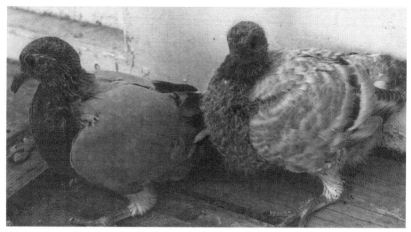

Youngsters showing the feather-grizzling resulting from paramyxovirus.

colour type, best seen at weaning but lost at the first moult.

- A similar phenomenon occurs in older birds where the ends of some body feathers develop an indistinct white area. It has a noticeable appearance because it develops mainly on the top of a pigeon's head. Pigeons displaying this white patch generally do not succeed at racing

5. Rare lesions of the eye include keratitis and blindness, occasionally seen in young birds.

Morbidity, mortality and stress

Morbidity is very high (90 – 100 %) and under normal conditions mortality is low (0 – 5 %). The mortality rate is closely linked to the amount of stress. Water deprivation has a profound effect on severely ill birds, causing mortality rates to rise dramatically.

It is imperative to cease breeding when stock birds are affected, as the raising of youngsters from 1 to 4 weeks is severely stressful. Failure to do so, results in increased mortality mainly owing to severe nephritis and internal gout. The squeakers that are raised are weak, poorly developed and do not develop into successful racers.

Racing stock showing signs of disease must be vaccinated and rested for two to three weeks. Mild circling during the lay-off period is permitted.

Pathology

Macroscopic changes are seen in the kidney with pale localised lesions, varying in size, to diffuse pale discolouration of the whole kidney. On occasion the kidneys must be removed from the carcase to examine the dorsal surface, which is otherwise not visible. Lesions are more easily detected in good light.

Following severe kidney damage, some pigeons die acutely with visceral gout. Urate crystals are deposited over the heart and other internal organs.

The pancreas may be affected, showing dark pink discolouration, with or without pale match-head size foci. Brain tissue may show congestion.

Microscopic changes are seen primarily in the kidney, which exhibits a varying degree of multifocal interstitial nephritis with lymphocytic and plasma cell infiltration. Epicardial necrosis and inflammation may be seen in heart tissue.

Diagnosis.

A diagnosis is usually made on the history and clinical picture. When the nervous system has been affected, paratyphoid must be ruled out by specific serological tests, or by culturing the organism. Confirmation of PMV infection in non-vaccinated birds, is done by positive H.I. studies. In vaccinated birds, virus isolation in embryonated chicken eggs is conclusive.

Treatment and control.

As with other virus diseases, there is no antiviral remedy. Paradoxical as it may seem, vaccination with inactivated vaccine shortens the period of polydipsa/polyuria. Within five to ten days of vaccination an improvement is seen in the droppings. Long-distance races have been won by birds vaccinated four weeks previously. Vaccination had no visible advantageous effect on birds showing nervous symptoms.

Scrupulous hygiene and regular disinfection of food and water containers with sodium hypochlorite is recommended. Multivitamin supplements are added to the drinking water and selected antibiotics are prescribed where necessary to control secondary infections.

Prophylactic vaccination is the only proper means of protection against the disease. Widely divergent opinions, paucity of controlled studies, and the general mistrust concerning vaccines, have resulted in an array of vaccines and vaccination schedules.

INACTIVATED VIRUS VACCINES

1. Oil emulsion heterologous ND vaccines eg. Newcadin, Newcavax (S. Africa), Newcavac, Chevivac and Paramyx 1 (no longer available), are used and proper controlled studies have shown these to be effective. Alexander & others demonstrated that two injections, four weeks apart, caused a strong immune response to develop (measured by HI tests). Vaccinated pigeons challenged by intravenous injection of a large dose of virulent PMV I virus (10 7.5 EID 50 of isolate 561/83) responded as follows: sick 1/10 and dead 1/10. This may seem to indicate a failure of protection, but the route is unusual and the quantity of dose is exceptionally high. Pigeons maintained under natural conditions are never likely to be challenged so severely. The same challenge dose administered to unvaccinated controls produced 100% mortality in all trials.

Vaccination with oil emulsion vaccine did not prevent birds from excreting virus up to 14 days after challenge, 21 days after vaccination.

Our experience is that inactivated ND vaccine is effective at a dose of 0.25 ml given subcutaneously, with two injections given four weeks apart with an optional further dose six months later, depending on the management, amount of stress (whether racing or breeding) and other extraneous factors. Much of our initial research into ND vaccine dosage was carried out before vaccines specifically licenced for racing pigeons were widely available. When using vaccines specifically designed for the racing pigeon market it is imperative that they use are used in accordance with the manufactuer's instructions. Indeed in some countries, the United Kingdom for example, it is the law that birds entered in races be vaccinated against PMV. In such circumstances it is foolish in the extreme, as well as illegal, to consider using any dosage other than that given by the manufacturer.

Our experience indicates that immunity is effective in controlling mortality and major symptoms but that complete protection is not gained. A subclinical disease situation occurs with stress producing symptoms. At autopsy small lesions are found in the kidney. Though the pigeon appears healthy, a bird subclinically infected with PMV, suffers from lack of endurance and form and becomes unable to carry off major honours.

2. Oil emulsion homologous vaccines have been produced in the U.S.A. but our knowledge of their effectivity is limited. An oil

emulsion vaccine containing homologous antigen has been developed and licensed in Europe (Nobivac Paramyxo). A full 12 month protection following a single vaccination is indicated in the product data sheet. There has been much debate about the relative merits of homologous verses heterologous vaccines, but there is no definitive published work comparing the two types of vaccines.

3. Carbomer adjuvant dead heterologous vaccine – water diluent. Only one vaccine of this type (Colombovac PMV) is commercially available. Yearlong protection is claimed with a single injection. "Both Nobivac Paramyxo and Colombovac PMV have been valuable additions to our armoury against Paramyxo infection in pigeons."

LIVE VIRUS VACCINES

1. La Sota ND vaccine.

First used in Belgium by Viaene & workers the vaccine has been used extensively in many countries – not always correctly. Through lack of understanding and incorrect advice, many fanciers have added the vaccine to the drinking water, with resultant failure of protection.

That administration of the vaccine to the drinking water does not provide sufficient protection, was borne out by practical results in France and Belgium and experimentally by Viaene & workers, who demonstrated nervous symptoms in four of thirteen pigeons, challenged six months after water vaccination. Viaene & workers showed that two doses of La Sota vaccine, administered 16 days apart, with a drop placed in each eye and nostril, resulted in a low level HI response but that all birds tested (15) fully resisted challenge to PMV I virus. The trials did not show for how long the protection persisted.

La Sota vaccine, correctly administered, provides strong, practical protection, though vaccinated birds are basketed for racing with pigeons from diseased lofts. Fears of shedding of vaccine virus and reversion to a virulent state have not been seen. Work by Dr.D. Senne of Ames, Iowa with smuggled live La Sota vaccine, showed no shedding and he was of the opinion that the vaccine virus does not replicate in pigeons.

It is illegal to import or use La Sota in some countries, including the United Kingdom which, apart from questions of the length of protection it offers, is a compelling reason to protect your pigeons with licensed inactivated vaccine.

2. In the Netherlands live La Sota vaccine virus has been injected subcutaneously by Van der Sluis. Duration of immunity was said to last six months and longer. No controlled experiments were done to support this contention and no obvious side-effects were recorded.

3. Hitchner B1 vaccine, produced very poor HI responses in trials by Alexander & workers. Vaccinated pigeons showed little resistance with 100% morbidity and 80% mortality. The use of Hitchner B1 vaccine as a preliminary procedure to using oil emulsion vaccine, showed no advantages. It therefore has no role to play in protecting pigeons against A/PMV 1

Summary of procedure;

During an outbreak

1. Cease all breeding and rearing activities.
2. Vaccinate all birds with inactivated vaccine according to manufacturer's instructions.
3. Give multivitamins as necessary.

In disease-free lofts two options are available:

1. Colombovac (or Nobivac) Paramyxo given once only and repeated yearly.
2. Where legal La Sota vaccine droplet method in eye and nose, given twice, one month apart and three-monthly thereafter.
3. Do not rely on Hitchner B1.

Outcome

Ineffective vaccination allows the symptoms to drag on for months. The position can be reversed with inactivated vaccine, correctly administered. Valuable birds showing nervous symptoms (including wing lameness) need not be destroyed: most will recover sufficiently for breeding purposes though recovery may take twelve months or longer.

3. Pigeon Pox

Pox in pigeons is caused by a viral infection and is characterised by discrete, proliferative lesions of the skin and/or mucuous membranes of the mouth and rarely the respiratory tract. The disease has a worldwide distribution and occurs regularly.

Etiology

Pox virus occurs in nearly all species of birds, 60 species having been recorded with naturally occurring pox infections and is seen frequently in wild doves. Although the disease is usually named after the host species, it would appear from the basic viral characteristics to be the same virus, albeit of different strains.

Transmission

The virus is transmitted by direct contact between infected and susceptible birds particularly when fighting, and indirectly by insect vectors such as mosquitoes and pigeon flies. Pox virus is found in saliva, which facilitates spread when pigeons peck each other, and in nasal and ocular discharges. From the saliva, drinking water is infected and spread rapidly occurs. The pox virus is unable to penetrate unbroken skin, but small abrasions allow infection, which fact is used when vaccination is performed.

Symptoms

Pigeon pox occurs in two forms; typical discrete wartlike pox

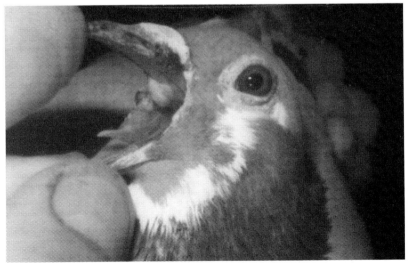

Pigeon Pox lesions on the wattles and inside the mouth.

lesions seen on the featherless parts of the skin, particularly the face, legs and feet and the diphtheritic form with moist yellow caseous, necrotic lesions in the mouth and, rarely, upper respiratory tract. Facial lesions in young and debilitated birds can become large and affect particularly the eyes, wattles and beak. In nestlings with an incomplete feather protection, pox lesions are found on all parts of the body, but in particular on the ear openings, wing butts and anus in addition to the usual sites.

The incubation period of the disease varies from four to fourteen days.

Pathogenesis

Infection with pox virus causes localised proliferation of epithelial cells. Affected cells become hyperplastic and hypertrophic. Large granular acidophilic intracytoplasmic inclusions (Bollinger's inclusion bodies) occur as the cells mature in the layers of epithelium. This "piling-up" of infected epithelial cells gives rise to the macroscopical pock formations.

Lesions are initially inflamed and haemorrhagic, they dessicate and form scabs which slough and allow new skin formation. A healthy adult pigeon with the skin form of pox can show lesions and be completely symptom-free within three weeks. The diphtheritic form takes longer as does the disease in young birds.

Secondary infections play an important role in aggravating pox injuries and the disease may then become life-threatening. Birds may lose an eye, toes or develope a skew beak. Many pigeons have one or both eyes permanently discoloured, a legacy of a pock on the lid with secondary infection in the eye.

Effect on Racing

With the pock formed and identified, there is little chance that any reasonable fancier would enter such an infected bird for racing, besides which most racing organisations would prohibit such an entry. It is, however, before lesions become visible that the disease is important.

Infected birds harbour the virus which is multiplying in the blood and bone marrow. In reaction to this invasion, the body develops a fever, which lasts for a few days, until the tissue reaction occurs and pox lesions appear. Except for some green droppings, this silent phase is missed by most fanciers, who may decide to enter these birds. This is hazardous. The pigeons are febrile, sick and should not be subjected to strenuous racing. Success is

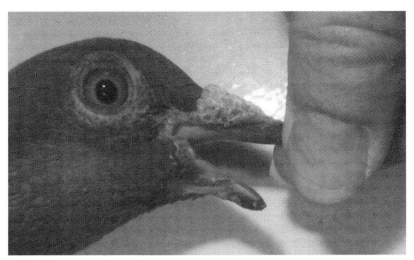

Severe Pigeon Pox left untreated, as will happen to feral birds, can result in permanent disfigurement, here the bird has lost one mandible (lower jaw).

not possible and should the race be difficult, valuable pigeons may be lost.

Once the pock has started to dry and the fever is gone, the pigeon can, theoretically, be raced. The lesions are localised and the results could be good. Such birds, however, are a threat to the other pigeons and should be refused participation. The virus is present in the dried-up scabs and very resistant, remaining active for months. Any fighting and pecking at the scabs could result in spread of the disease.

Diagnosis

Though diagnosed quite readily from the typical lesions, early cases may present difficulties. Histopathological examination, demonstrating intracytoplasmic Bollinger bodies, is regarded as conclusive. Diagnosis in a bird is aided by an examination of the loftmates for signs of typical lesions. If these are found, it must be assumed that pox is present in the other birds, not yet showing symptms.

Pox lesions are differentiated from the following disorders.

1. In the early stages a pox lesion developing on an eyelid, may

resemble vitamin A deficiency, mild ornithosis (one-eye cold), a peck on the eyelid or non-specific conjuntivitis..

2. The diphtheritic form of pox is easily confused with oral trichomoniasis (crop canker). Pox lesions are difficult to remove from the mucous membrane, being fleshy, covered with a yellow exudate and firmly attached. They are found in the anterior part of the mouth, and bleed profusely if forcibly removed. Canker lesions occur more in the back of the throat, are cheesy in substance and readily removed.

Treatment

No effective treatment exists against pox. Local applications of disinfectants or antibiotics will help control secondary infections, and appear to shorten the course of the disease. Iodine solutions and tinctures are usually employed for this purpose. Young birds can be severely affected; eg. with a closed, swollen and purulent eye, a mutilated beak etc. and it is my opinion that such birds are better culled. Individual treatment may be given to valuable future stock, as their breeding potential is not affected.

Control

Concurrent problems such as coccidiosis and crop canker should be controlled to reduce the stress on young birds. The resistance of the pigeons is stimulated by the addition of vitamins to the food or water. Additional sources of vitamin A are unnecessary, but the addition of vitamins of the B complex and E is beneficial.

Vaccination for pigeon pox provides effective protection. For best results this is done twice in six weeks, with yearly boosters. With the prevalence of natural pox, I have found a single vaccination to be sufficient, provided that it "grows". Although not essential to do older birds, I use a routine whereby all the race birds in the loft are done once a year, and find it satisfactory.

Vaccines such as Nobivac Pigeon Pox vaccine and the one manufactured by the State Veterinary Laboratories at Onderstepoort, South Africa, are effective, cheap and easy to use. They are completely safe and will in no way affect the future racing ability of the pigeons.

Precaution

It is imperative that the vaccine, which is a freeze-dried product, be handled correctly. Failure to do so results in a failed vaccination, necessitating revaccination and having pigeons that are at risk.

It is a live biological product with a limited life and the expiry date must be honoured. Do not use expired stock. Before use, the vaccine must be kept refrigerated at 4 degrees C and the vaccine must be kept out of direct sunlight at all times.
   Once reconstituted, the vaccine must be used within an hour. It cannot be kept, even refrigerated, till the next day.

Method

One of two popular methods is used.

A. A few feathers (5 to 10) are plucked from the upper leg and the reconstituted vaccine is applied with a small hard brush to the exposed feather follicles. Vigorous application will ensure good penetration of the vaccine.

B. With a needle dipped in the liquid vaccine, a scratch is made through the skin on the exposed breast. The method is quicker but frowned upon by some authorities as being too close to the major flight muscles, the powerhouse of the pigeon.

After five days the vaccinated area begins to swell and a typical pox lesion develops. This has usually dried and fallen off, twelve to fourteen days later, completing the procedure. Should no "growth" take place, the vaccination has failed in which instance it may have to be repeated.

Some reasons for possible failure are;

1. Vaccine was old; check expiry date.
2. Vaccine stored at wrong temperature, (kept in a hot car?)
3. Vaccine exposed to direct sunlight.
4. Vaccine used too long after reconstitution (mixed morning, used afternoon?)
5. Vaccine incorrectly applied and did not penetrate broken skin.
6. Pigeons already immune; either from previous vaccination or natural exposure. (Natural exposure can occur unnoticed by the fancier as some pox lesions are small and insignificant.)

In-season infection

Besides the odd bird that develops serious pox, the disease is not a problem during the off-season. Healthy birds with pox lesions may be left alone as they will recover quickly and acquire a strong immunity.

During the racing season, however, the appearance of pox can spoil many plans and should infection arise, a few procedures may be adopted.

1. If the majority of pigeons are immune and only the few susceptible birds develop pox, little is done. The affected birds are teporarily withdrawn from the race team, allowed to recover and rejoin the team a month later.

2. All the racers are susceptible. The team is divided into two halves, one of which is vaccinated. These birds are not raced or trained, although circling is continued. As soon as the vaccination scabs have dropped off, this half resumes racing and the process is repeated with the other half which has, in the meanwhile, continued racing. A danger exists in that pigeons in the incubation phase of the disease are not recognised and sent on long-distance races.

2. Racing is ceased altogether (unless there are immune pigeons from previous years) and all pigeons are vaccinated. Racing resumes when the birds have lost their vaccination scabs.

4. Pigeon Herpesvirus (PHV)

Generally unknown and not readily recognised, pigeon herpesvirus (PHV) nevertheless frequently occurs. Mostly mistaken for crop canker, sick birds are rapidly culled and as the disease is self-limiting, it is forgotten once the outbreak has cleared. Variation in susceptibility is seen, with all birds not visibly affected, the majority having a subclinical infection.

The disease has been recognized in the USA, Australasia, many European countries and Africa, where the virus was positively identified by Pollard & Marais. To date all herpesvirus isolates from pigeons have shown the same antigenic and cultural properties.

A serological survey to determine the frequency of virus infections in pigeons revealed that 63% of 75 pigeons tested, were positive for herpesvirus antibodies. This seems to indicate that many lofts harbour infected birds.

Symptoms

Two disease syndromes were thought to occur. True herpesvirus affects the upper digestive tract, whereas the other form, attacking

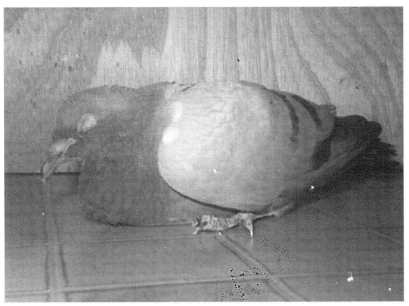

Typical pose of a youngster affected by Pigeon Herpesvirus. The bird appears sleepy, sits hunched up and does not move. Once this stage is reached, mortality occurs.

the nervous system, has been shown to be a variant avian paramyxovirus type 1. Failing to respond to the standard treatments, the chronic form is a perplexing and demoralising condition for the fancier to deal with.

In the acute form, the usual symptoms seen are those of general weakness, depression, anorexia, nasal discharge, dirty wattles and the accumulation of a yellowish exudate in the mouth, throat and pharynx. Clinical signs and lesions vary markedly in their severity. Seriously affected birds are usually less than six months old. An affected bird rapidly loses weight, becomes very depressed and death occurs four to six day after the first symptoms were

observed. Severe depression is the striking feature of the symptoms. Affected birds refuse food and water and are unwilling to
move about when chased, creating an impression of extreme
sleepiness.

The chronic form occurs in adult, actively racing pigeons, in
whom nothing is seen, other than an inexplicable loss of condition.
Difficulty in swallowing has been noted.

Pathology

In the acute form the rotten stench that emanates from the
necrotic and affected parts, is immediately apparent when the bird
is opened for autopsy. Mild inflammation is seen of the mouth,
pharynx, oesophagus and crop with affected parts thinly covered
with a layer of whitish-creamy non-adherent exudate, particularly
in the oesophagus and crop. The liver is enlarged and pale, with
white foci 0.2 mm in diameter.

Histopathology of the liver reveals focal necrotic hepatitis with
basophilic and eosinophillic intranuclear inclusions. The crop and
oesophagus show vacuolar and cellular degeneration of the epithelium. Small ulcers are seen in some areas, and intranuclear inclusions are seen in the epithelial cells in and surrounding the
lesions.

The chronic form of the disease is regognised by the accumulation of creamy non-adherent exudate in the crop. Microscopical
examination is negative.

Diagnosis

The disease is suspected from the clinical picture and autopsy, and
confirmed by histology, (the presence of intranuclear inclusions is
conclusive) or virus isolation.

Herpesvirus infection must be differentiated from trichomoniasis
(demonstration of parasites in a throat swab), ornithosis (intranuclear inclusion bodies in a swab of the ocular mucous membrane or
positive IFA test), and tuberculosis and paratyphoid (serology or
bacterial culture). Care must be exercised when PHV and cropcanker occur simultaneously (commonly).

Should the symptoms and pathology exist in the absence of cropcanker, chronic PHV must be suspected.

Treatment and Control

There is no effective treatment. Nevertheless control of the disease includes; immediate removal of affected pigeons, disinfection of premises and utensils, strict hygiene regarding the feeding and watering practices, administration of antibiotics to control secondary infections and vitamins to help support against stress.

Chlorine-based derivatives (Milton, Halamid etc.) are recommended for disinfection purposes.

It has been observed that treatment for trichomoniasis is ineffective when PHV is present.

5. Arbovirus

Although the arboviruses have not, to my knowledge, been isolated outside the USA, their emergence, with relaxed importation laws in some countries, is theoretically possible. The virus occurs endemically in many species of American birds, from whence it has spread to pigeons. The main reason for the bird import embargo from the USA into South Africa, is the danger of disease to the local horse population, which is very susceptible to the virus. (Arboviruses cause Equine encephalitis in horses).

As the practical implications of arbovirus introductions do affect us, a brief review of the relevant literature follows.

Etiology and Transmission

Several species of mosquitoes serve as biological vectors for the virus. Control of the virus depends to a large extent therefore on controlling the mosquito population.

Symptoms

Symptoms exhibited by pigeons, relate to the degree of affectation of the nervous system; loss of balance, inability to drink leading to depression, paralysis and abnormal postures of the head and neck. Tremors may be seen and torticollis is a common sign. Many cases end in severe depression, coma and death. (Symptoms are similar paramyxovirosis, neurological form)

Pathology

The major lesions are those of a non-suppurative encephalitis. However the findings are non-specific and of little diagnostic value.

Diagnosis

The diagnosis is based on isolation and identification of the virus, or demonstration of specific antibodies in the serum.

Treatment and Control

No treatment is available and control consists of breaking the life-cycle of the virus by eradication of the vector mosquitoes.

6. Adenovirus

History

Adenovirus has long been recognised as a cause of enteritis with loose, stinking motions in young pigeons. The appearance is acute, the disease has a low mortality, and spontaneous recovery occurs. During the years 1991-1992, clinical symptoms resulting from pathology of the digestive and respiratory systems and characterised by green, foul-smelling droppings, were seen in racing pigeons in South Africa. Eventually an adenovirus and an E. coli, were isolated from samples of pigeon material. More recently the disease has been reported in Great Britain, initially in the North East and then elsewhere during 1994 and 1995.
    A survey carried out in Belgium to determine the relative frequency of virus infections in pigeons, revealed that 3% of 75 pigeons tested, were positive for antibodies. This seems to suggest that the disease is not commonly present.

Transmission

Virus is found in the faecal and respiratory excretions and transmission occurs via contaminated food and water and by direct contact.

Symptoms

Adenovirus, widespread around the world, was reckoned to be a disease of young birds, occurring in isolated cases only. It occurred sporadically but in the latest outbreaks, many lofts were affected intermittently over two years. Symptoms vary, but include;

  - Foul-smelling, bright green excreta

- Vomiting
- Loss of condition
- Variable respiratory symptoms
- Mortalities, 0-20%
- Poor race results
- Increased losses from races

Recovered birds can remain carriers and show the following symptoms;

- Intermittent diarrhoea
- Poor race results and poor returns with many pigeons lost
- Decreased resistance to other diseases

Pathology

Except for a mild enteritis (which may be present in the absence of diarrhoea), no macroscopical changes constantly occur. In severe cases changes are seen in the liver, intestine, lungs and kidneys. Microscopically, intranuclear inclusions are seen in liver and intestinal cells. (To increase the chances of finding inclusions, samples are preferably taken from a fresh carcase.)

Diagnosis

The diagnosis is made on demonstrating the typical intranuclear inclusion bodies in liver or intestinal cells or by demonstrating the organism with electronmicroscopy in faeces material. The disease must be differentiated from hexamitiasis, paramyxovirosis, paratyphoid, poisoning and herpes virus infection.

Discussion

Usually, when adenovirus causes pathology, it has been found in association with E. coli, a bacteria which belongs to the normal gut flora and which can be pathogenic or not. E. coli found with adenovirus in the past has not been pathogenic. As adenovirus is not normally pathogenic to adult pigeons, synergism between the virus and the bacteria is thought to occur, leading to acute disease and mortality in susceptible birds. Though synergism is as yet unproven, we accept it as fact and treat accordingly.

Treatment and Control

There is no effective treatment for adenovirus. E. coli, however can
be treated with many antibiotics including cloramphenicol, potentiated sulphonamides, enrofloxacin (Baytril), danofloxacin (Avocin)
etc. Multivitamin supplementation to reduce the effect of stress
and high doses of vitamins C and E, help to boost resistance.

7. Ornithosis

Chlamydial infections have been isolated from 140 species of wild
birds, with the feral city pigeon (Columbia livia) as a common and
consistent source of infection. Chlamydia organisms cause psittacosis, a highly contagious disease of the parrot family and
ornithosis in other birds and pigeons. Man contracts fatal psittacosis from parrots and ornithosis, which is less serious, from other
birds.
    Chlamydias are grouped with the larger viruses, though they
possess some properties of bacteria, amongst which is susceptibility to certain antibiotics.

Etiology

Chlamydia psittaci is the cause of the disease in birds, and many
strains, varying in pathogenicity, have been isolated. Different
strains affect mammals, causing abortion, pneumonitis, arthritis,
encephalitis or conjunctivitis.
    Chlamydia psittaci in man, causes a severe pneumonitis, accom-
panied by headache and dizziness, the occurrence of which in a
pigeon or psittacine owner, must be regarded as a serious warning
signal for further investigation.
    Some authors believe the condition in pigeons to be a complex of
diseases, the 'ornithosis complex' and that chlamydias acting with
mycoplasmas, haemophilus, E. coli and other organisms, are
responsible for the classical syndrome. We are of the opinion that
Chlamydia alone can cause symptoms. Pigeons can be asympto-
matic carriers.
    Certain European authorities believe that the symptoms seen in
so-called ornithosis, may be linked to incorrect loft ventilation.
Draughts are blamed for a variety of syndromes, e.g. "one eye
cold". Ideally a loft is closed, with a maximum occupation rate of
two pigeons per cubic metre. In South Africa most lofts are over-
crowded and have many times that number.

Transmission

The virus is transmitted via the faeces and nasal discharges of infected birds. Pigeons in inadequate housing, particularly with poor ventilation and overcrowding, are more likely to contract the disease. Racing and training baskets provide ideal conditions for the spread of chlamydia.

Symptoms

The symptoms associated with this complex condition are variable. In adult birds the first sign is a reluctance of the pigeons to fly. The eyes are affected, the eyelids swell slightly and the corneas become moist. The infected eye is irritating to the bird, scratched with a foot or rubbed on the shoulder and a wet patch appears on the wing. The changes in the eyes are often unilateral, causing the familiar "one eye cold". The wattles are slightly moist and discoloured, discharges increase, become purulent and cause the eyelids to stick together. Keratitis of the eye, discolouring the iris, follows. The nasal discharges remain watery or become purulent with the birds sneezing frequently. With a purulent exudate the pigeons shake their heads, spattering exudate all round them. Sneezing may occur without a noticeable nasal discharge and may be the only sign of ornithosis.

The mucous membranes of the mouth and throat, normally a rosy colour, become blueish. The edges of the larynx are swollen and the epiglottis opens and closes indicating that breathing is pronounced and laboured. The opening in the palate may be closed by the swollen edges.

Characteristic of ornithosis is the pronounced respiratory rales, heard at each breath and caused by pus and exudate in the trachea and airsacs. Flying vigour is reduced, appetite diminished and the birds are obviously ill. The skin over the pectoral muscles loses its rosy colour becoming blueish and scurfy. The birds have loose, green droppings and rapidly lose condition.

Mortality in old birds is low, young birds are more susceptible. Nest babies may die acutely. Young birds will progress rapidly through many if not all the various symptoms, whereas older birds may show only one symptom per pigeon.

Adult pigeons can make a good recovery and go on to become successful racers, consequently it is unwise to destroy sick birds at the first sign. Relapses do occur, however, and one must eliminate carriers.

Usually only a few birds are affected at a time. When these have cleared a few more are affected, the process repeating itself until the infection fades naturally. Under stressful conditions, however, relapses may occur, and during the racing season this could be disastrous, as the birds struggle to maintain condition and when raced, come late or are lost.

Pathogenesis

A distinction is made between old birds with the chronic form and young birds which usually show acute symptoms.

Young birds of two to four weeks of age are most susceptible. Within four to 15 days after infection they develop diarrhoea, rapidly lose condition, become emaciated and die. Chlamydias damage mainly the liver, spleen and bonemarrow.

Not all birds are severely affected. Loss of form and poor racing results, may be the only indication of infection. From a racing aspect the chronic form is more serious because of the difficulty of diagnosis. The main effects of chronic infection are liver degeneration, resulting in a fatty liver, and permanent lung and heart damage. Recovered pigeons of both the acute and chronic forms may become symptomless carriers and serve as a source of infection for loftmates.

Pathology

Tremendous variation in the degree of pathology exists, depending on the age and resistance of the individual bird. Stress, caused by concurrent diseases such as mycoplasmosis, coccidiosis, trichomoniasis, worms or other debilitating conditions, decreases individual resistance.

Macroscopic lesions are mainly found in the liver, spleen and pericardium. We see pseudomembranous peritonitis over the serosal surfaces, enlargement of the liver with a mottled appearance and a greatly enlarged black spleen. The heart is enlarged in chronic cases.

Microscopically we find most changes in the liver, where proliferation of lymphoid tissue around the bileducts eventuates in compression of the ducts, plugging, necrosis and rupture with hepatic cell necrosis. Haemosiderosis is seen in both the liver and spleen.

Diagnosis

The symptoms of "one eye cold", poor performance and loss of condition in mature birds is strongly suspicious. Laboratory tests to confirm the disease consist of a biological test (in mice, guinea pigs or embryonated eggs), serology (direct complement fixation test, and IFA test), and histopathology (presence of elementary bodies in impression smears of the conjunctiva, liver and spleen, stained by Stamp's method).

Differential diagnoses

Because the disease is regarded as an ornithosis-complex rather than as a specific entity, there are few conditions with which it may be confused.
1. Beaking young adult hens may develop wet-discoloured wattles particularly early in the season. Careful observation will distinguish this from a disease condition.

2. Pigeons feeding babies develop a brownish discolouration on the sides of the wattles. Careful observation will recognise this and allow for distinction from the diseased state.

3. Mycoplasmosis. Mycoplasmas are regarded by Schrag to be capable of causing disease on their own. Most authorities are of the opinion that they do not act independently to cause disease, probably occurring together with the chlamydias in respiratory diseases, where either one is diagnosed.
   (We believe that the mycoplasmas, acting alone, do not cause overt disease but play an important role in affecting performance. In combination with other organisms, they can cause disease.)

Prognosis

Ornithosis spreads slowly in a loft and though symptoms are not readily seen in all the birds, the majority are infected. Recovery in strong, healthy pigeons is good, with little or no sign of lasting infection. Carriers do occur and continue to shed infective particles, particularly in the droppings. To eradicate the disease from a loft, the carriers must be identified and eliminated.

Treatment and Control

Most healthy, strong pigeons will recover from ornithosis without treatment and the disease could be left to run its course. This could take weeks or months and an outbreak during the racing season could not be handled in this manner, as racing is handicapped till recovery occurs. Treatment, on the other hand, is effective and speeds recovery.

A combination of antibiotics (eg.tylosine + chlortetracycline or spiramycine + oxytetracycline), has been found to be effective. Injections of streptomycin or tylosine may be given in individual cases.

The use of streptomycin is interesting; Stam found that chlamydias were not susceptible to streptomycin, in spite of which, marked improvement resulted from the use of the drug. In addition it was found that the more severe the toxic reaction to the injection, which varied from vomiting to total loss of consciousness, the quicker the recovery; so much so that that some birds were in prize-winning form within days following treatment.

It is a debatable issue whether a loft should be sterilised of chlamydias prior to the racing season. Prolonged treatment is required and close contact in the racing panniers would soon cause re-infection. Our recommendation is that preventative treatment is not given and that control is aimed at keeping concurrent debilitating conditions at a minimum. Healthy pigeons' natural resistance will protect them against with chlamydia. Upon outbreak of symptoms, effective antibiotics can be used to combat the disease.

8. Ulcerative Enteritis of Pigeons (UEP)

To include UEP under the viruses is somewhat presumptive and not fully scientifically answerable. However, it has been included here because all the indications point to a viral etiology and it has occurred with such stubborn regularity over the past few years that it has become a realistic entity. I have been unable able to find a description of this condition but should future knowledge identify it as part of an already established disease or as a hitherto undescribed one, at least some attention shall have been drawn to the condition.

History

UEP first became came to our knowledge in 1980, when it suddenly appeared in South Africa and within weeks moved through a zone, 100 km wide. The affected pigeons belonged to fanciers of separate clubs and separate unions, and were transported to races on two different vehicles.

The disease first appeared during the racing season and the race results of affected pigeons deteriorated drastically. From thereon sporadic outbreaks occurred and the disease has not re-appeared on a large scale since.

Etiology

The cause is unknown, suspected of being a virus. Bacterial studies have not given any indication except in one case when a pathogenic E. coli (type O124:K72 {B17}) was isolated. The rapid spread, resistance to well-known antibiotics, microscopic pathology and self-limitation in a loft, corroborate the belief that a virus is the primary pathogen. Transmission within a loft probably takes place via contamination of the food and water with faeces.

Symptoms

All affected birds have been younger than three years, mostly yearlings or young birds, seeming to indicate that older birds are more resistant, possibly having built up immunity following subclinical infection. I have not seen nestlings with the disease.

The signs are those of any enteritis. The birds pass loose, sloppy droppings, lose condition and fail to do well in races. Newly-weaned youngsters lose weight to an extreme degree, rapidly becoming emaciated and weak. Older birds appear to be reasonably well and show loss of condition only on being handled. Some birds show signs of respiratory distress, breathing with an open mouth.

Pathology

On autopsy the carcase is thin and slightly dehydrated. In uncomplicated cases the intestine is the only affected organ. Small raised circular areas, 4 to 5 mm in diameter, are seen on the peritoneal lining (serosa) of the bowel. They are found either in the anterior (duodenal) and middle segment, or in the posterior part (colon) of the intestine. The mucosal surface reveals small discreet ulcers with a raised circumference.

Secondary infection is common, affecting particularly the airsacs, which are coated with a thin yellowish exudate. In more advanced cases, secondary aspergillosis is common.

Microscopically the mucosa is thickened by infiltration of inflammatory cells, consisting mainly of lymphocytes and pseudo-eosinophils and proliferation of the epithelium particularly in the crypts of Lieberkuhn. Basophilic intranuclear inclusion bodies have been found in the epithelial cells, in some cases. Cellular infiltration is seen in the mesentery, and as nests of cells in the circular and longitudinal muscle layers of the intestine.

Diagnosis

The diagnosis is established on autopsy. The disease must be distinguished from paratyphoid, adenovirosis, capillariasis, hexamitiasis and non-specific enteritides.

Treatment and Control

No treatment at present is effective, but suitable antibiotics (eg. chloramphenicol, trimethoprim etc.) seem to shorten the course of the disease, probably because the antibiotics contain secondary invaders. The pigeon's defense mechanisms develop immunity to the virus and the disease gradually subsides.

Regular and thorough disinfection with sodium hypochlorite and scrupulous hygiene are essential. Food and water must at all times be protected from contamination with faeces.

Chapter 5

Bacterial and Mycotic diseases

1. Paratyphoid

Paratyphoid is one form of salmonellosis, a condition caused by the Salmonella group of bacteria of which more than 1100 have been identified. The group was named after Dr. Salmon an American veterinarian who first described and identified the disease.

Paratyphoid in pigeons is caused by Salmonella typhimurium. It is one of the most widely occurring diseases of pigeons and is arguably one of the most important.

Baay found that in the Netherlands 5% of the lofts and 28% of the racing baskets at the start of the racing season, rising to 67% at the end of the season, were infected with paratyphoid.

The disease appears even in the most meticulously kept and clean establishment and upon investigation, it may be found to be widespread and deeply rooted, requiring a concerted effort for its eradication. Serious losses occur, with high mortality in young birds, while many old birds have to be destroyed.

Etiology.

Salmonella typhimurium var. copenhagen (with antigen structure O:1,4,12;H:i,1,2.) is the specific pathogen causing paratyphoid in pigeons. Phage-typing disclosed that types 2 and 690 were involved in more that 90% of cases. Other salmonellae have been found in pigeons eg. S. abortus equi and S. dublin rough, but these are rare and of little consequence.

Rodents, particularly rats and mice, are well-known carriers of salmonellae, including S. typhimurium. Rodent eradication from and around the loft is obligatory if one is to establish a disease-free loft of pigeons.

It has been found that S. typhimurium is not a factor in the epidemiology of human salmonellosis.

Symptoms.

The clinical picture of paratyphoid in pigeons varies considerably and five main symptom complexes, subdivided through their locality expression, are found. More than one form of the disease is often seen together.

1. Enteric form.

Salmonellae are classified under the enterobacteria and are nearly always found in the gut and faeces.

In older birds the enteric form of the disease may remain unnoticed for weeks or months. The droppings be completely normal and the birds show no symptoms at all.

Exceptional cases are on record where infected pigeons have raced well and have scored winning positions. Only bacterial culture of the droppings and serum antibody neutralisation tests (less specific) can identify these birds.

As a rule, however, infected pigeons do not come into condition. They lose weight dramatically and often the faeces are slimy and green with bubbles. The differential diagnoses include all other causes of enteritis including endoparasites. Every pigeon losing condition in the absence of worm infestation is suspect for paratyphoid.

Squeakers and babies in the nest are severely affected. Diarrhoea is seen with faeces coating the vent-feathers. Rapid loss of condition follows and a high percentage of acute mortalities occurs.

2. Articular form.

This form of the disease occurs in both young and old pigeons. The organisms enter the system orally, multiply in the intestine and localise in one or more of the joints. The elbow joint of the wing is the most common site.

Sometimes the first indication that an adult pigeon has contracted paratyphoid is a slight lopsidedness in flight. On closer examination, the joint is obviously swollen, hot and painful and the wing droops. Following incision a clear, mucoid, straw-coloured fluid escapes from the swelling. In an acute case the joint fluid can be red-tinged. The affected joint progressively causes more interference with flying till eventually the bird is unable to use the wing, which droops and becomes frayed, tattered and dirty. Such a bird will not recover and it is preferable to cull is as a it remains a threat to the health of the remaining birds.

Differential diagnoses of wing lameness include:

- Post-laying weakness in hens which usually corrects itself in a few days. The bird is too weak to stand or fly and the condition is prevented by calcium supplementation.

- Fracture or dislocation of the wing. A broken bone in the wing will allow excessive movement and grating is heard, whereas a dislocated joint limits the mobility of the wing, putting the joint under tension.

- Localised haemorrhages, bruising or wounds. Careful examination will reveal the true situation.

Leg lameness occurs as result of pain in the toes, foot or upper leg but mostly in the hock joint. If present in both legs, the pigeon will find it very difficult to stand and will mostly rest on his hocks.
    The condition must be differentiated from gout, fractures, bumblefoot, and a tight metal ring, causing obstruction to the flow of blood with swelling, pain and eventually gangrene.

3. Nervous form.

Salmonellae readily enter the nervous tissue of the brain especially the cerebellum, causing loss of balance, torticollis (twisting of the neck) and other bizarre reactions. Most often the pigeon is seen, lying on its breastbone with the neck twisted and gazing upwards (stargazers).
    Abnormal movements include continuous circular movements of the head and neck, head held to one side, head held forward and down between the legs or pulled back between the shoulders so far that the bird falls over backwards or convulsions.
    The nervous form of paratyphoid is differentiated from all types of poisoning, vitamin deficiency especially vitamin B1, paramyxovirus and toxoplasmosis.

4. Internal form.

This form of the disease includes any of the forms mentioned earlier and is possibly the most serious. Usually all the internal organs are affected. Young birds develop septicaemia with severe diarrhoea. They are listless, droopy, short of breath and die rapidly. Older birds are more resistant, developing chronic disease with severe wasting of the tissues.

A pure culture of S. typhimurium can usually be cultured from the liver which is swollen and discoloured pale yellow or dark green-black.

Ocasionally small subcutaneous abscesses develop which, when cultured, yield salmonellae eg. below the lower eyelids.

The internal form is seen on rare occasions as a unilateral panopthalmia.

5. Reproductive form.

The reproductive form is usually classified under the internal form. We make a distinction because sometimes it is the first or only obvious sign of paratyphoid in a loft. Three scenarios are possible:

- In the hen salmonellae may localise in the ovary, with the following possibilities. Infected eggs result in the death of the embryos before the tenth day of hatching or with advanced ovarian infection, regression of the ova takes place and the hen becomes permanently sterile.

- Faecal contamination of the egg allows the motile bacteria to penetrate the eggshell and infect the developing embryo. The chipped egg fails to hatch with the baby dying in the shell or soon after chipping out.

- In the cock the testes are infected, rendering the pigeon sterile. Normal eggs are laid by the hen but fail to develop. The sterility is generally permanent.

When these breeding problems arise the fancier is well advised to have his stock birds tested for paratyphoid, even though no other obvious signs of the disease are apparent.

Pathogenesis

The incubation period after infection is about four to five days. The organisms multiply in the gut and enter the bloodstream causing septicaemia.

In young and debilitated older pigeons, the organisms rapidly multiply in the body and cause acute mortality.

In strong older birds the disease is chronic and a long drawn-out course is characteristic. The pigeons contract the enteric, articular and reproductive forms of the disease and few birds die as an immediate result. The birds that contract the nervous form, with brain lesions, invariably do not survive.

Pigeons that survive the chronic disease and do not receive adequate treatment often become carriers, continue to excrete organisms in the faeces or eggs and establish a permanent cycle of the disease.

Pathology

In parallel with the symptoms, autopsy changes are variable. In some of the less severe, more chronic forms, no pathological changes are evident.

The internal form usually shows the most changes with nearly all organs affected. Internal abscessation is a standard finding. The liver, spleen and kidneys are severely swollen. The kidneys are lighter in colour and have a mottled dirty-cream appearance. Creamy-grey abscesses of various size may be seen in the liver, lungs and musculature.

The colour of the liver may be dark and blackish or lighter than normal with necrotic foci. The intestine shows haemorrhagic enteritis with multiple small yellowish-white spots of necrosis and ulcerations or single discrete ulcers.

Large inspissated abscesses are found in the oviduct, often in association with ovarian abscesses and necrosis of the ova.

Diagnosis

A diagnosis is made from the history, clinical symptoms, autopsy and laboratory findings. Any history of poor hatchability or nestling mortality is suspicious. In the absence of verminosis, paratyphoid is suspected in all cases of chronic wasting. Diarrhoea with wing and/or leg lameness coupled with poor growth and stunting is strongly indicative. An autopsy is supportive and laboratory findings are definitive:

- The droppings of sick pigeons are repeatedly cultured for the presence of salmonellae. One negative result is not significant and the test must be repeated three times at weekly intervals before a final opinion can be expressed.

- If the birds have not been vaccinated, a serum agglutination test can indicate the presence of antibodies. A positive test means that the pigeon has had the disease and is recovered, or is harbouring the infection and is possibly excreting organisms.

Young, recently infected or very debilitated birds may give a false negative test. Any pigeon vaccinated up to one year before testing may have circulating vaccine antibodies which results in a false positive test. At present the test reagent is not available throughout the world.

Treatment and control

There is at present no adequate (100% effective) treatment. Good results are achieved by using antibiotics (chloramphenicol, oxytetracycline, ampicillin) in combination with chemotherapeutics (furoxone and furazolidone). Concurrent medication with vitamin B complex is recommended. Carriers persist.

The birds that have joint disease for more than four days or chronic symptoms of torticollis and emaciation, will not recover and should be culled. Swollen joints are not responsive to treatment (draining of the joint results in refilling within 24 hours) and invariably become ankylosed. Cortisone treatment is not preventive.

There is at present no acceptably efficient vaccine. Not one of five commercially-available vaccines, tested by Ruger & Raddei (1978) could prevent increased serum titres, salmonella excretion or recovery of salmonella from various organs, following experimental challenge. All available vaccines provided a reasonable immunity for 6 to 8 months – giving enough protection against most levels of natural exposure.

Control is multi-faceted; The following routine is recommended.

1. Treatment with an antibiotic/chemotherapeutic/vitamin mixture for two weeks.

2. Disinfection of all premises and utensils with a suitable disinfectant. The use of a chlorine-based product is advisable.

3. Culling of all birds chronically thin, sterile, or with ankylosed joints and eradication of all birds excreting positive faeces – any one of three samples, tested one week apart.

4. Vaccination of the remaining pigeons. The vaccine (not available

throughout the world) consists of inactivated (killed) paratyphoid bacteria and may precipitate an attack upon administration, if the pigeon is already infected. All reactors are removed.

5. Young birds are vaccinated a second time, three to four weeks later. Vaccines against pox, paramyxovirus and paratyphoid, may be given simultaneously.

6. If possible, the source of the infection is traced and eliminated.

2. Mycoplasmosis

Mycoplasmas occur worldwide in a wide variety of species and produce many differing disease conditions. In poultry they cause respiratory diseases, viz. infectious sinusitis in turkeys and chronic respiratory disease (CRD) in chickens.

Although various mycoplasmas have been isolated from the respiratory tract of pigeons, most authorities are agreed that they are not primary pathogens and do not, by themselves, cause disease. Viaene found that mycoplasmas when introduced into healthy pigeons did not produce disease. Mycoplasmas isolated from sick pigeons are found in conjunction with other disease processes, such as ornithosis, paratyphoid etc. Schrag considered that the organisms on their own are capable of producing disease.

For pigeon fanciers, mycoplasma is serious, even though no scientific evidence of their pathocenicity exists. It is believed that the organisms predipose the pigeon to other respiratory infections, particularly ornithosis and E. coli. More importantly, mycoplasmosis is regarded as an erosion disease i.e., pigeons, though appearing healthy, cannot have super health if they harbour mycoplasma organisms and are prevented from achieving top racing results.

Etiology and Transmission

Mycoplasmas are small (120 to 500 mu) pleomorphic organisms, which colour blue with Giemsa stain. They are fairly labile and can survive only one week outside the host. According to Schrag, all pigeons must be considered to be infected.

Transmission occurs via faecal contamination of food and water, droplet infection from eye, nose and oral discharges, and from direct handling. In the race basket, with the inevitable close contact and communal drinking facilities, spread of the organism becomes unavoidable. The incubation period is relatively long, 10 to 24 days, with the result that the effect of a new introduction into the loft, spreads relatively slowly.

Symptoms

According to Schrag, a watery nasal discharge, which becomes more slimy-pussy is the first indication. This colours the wattles, causing the sick birds to be identified easily. We have not seen this first step.

Slime is seen in the throat and threads of slime are seen from the tongue to the roof of the mouth. The mucus membranes of the throat and mouth are inflamed and swollen.

Pressure on the wattles may elicit a slimy discharge. At night with the birds at rest, a gurgling sound is heard because of inflamed and semi-blocked airways.

Schrag maintains that the only symptom of chronic mycoplasmosis is seen in deteriorating performances. We have found the same. Short races exhaust the birds. They are unwilling to fly and do so with difficulty. Circling around the loft is stressful and affected birds cease flying after a few minutes, dropping onto the loft or nearest rooftop.

Course of the disease

A long drawn-out course is typical. The airsacs become inflamed, are attacked by secondary bacterial invaders and coated with a purulent exudate. This prevents the airsacs from fulfilling their function, and any exertion becomes difficult and stressful. With poor blood supply to the airsacs, the aerocystitis is resistant to treatment, causing chronic respiratory disease and leaving the pigeon useless for racing. It is advisable to cull all pigeons that do not respond to treatment.

Diagnosis

Mycoplasmas can be cultured in the laboratory but require special tests for identification and few institutions are equipped or willing to this for pigeons. Serological tests for mycoplasmosis are widely used in the poultry industry and could be developed for pigeons if the demand were strong enough.

Diagnosis on the live bird is complicated by concurrent infections, particularly ornithosis, aspergillosis and E. coli.

Ornithosis is a serious and acute disease masking the symptoms of mycoplasmosis. Mortalities occur in young birds, while old birds show obvious signs such as swollen, inflamed eyelids, purulent nasal discharge and respiratory distress. If treatment for ornithosis fails to bring about improvement, the presence of mycoplasmosis must be considered.

Aspergillosis causes respiratory distress with reluctance to fly but the mouth, throat and nose will be clear, with lesions confined to the lungs and airsacs.

Treatment

Antibiotics are successful, particularly in the earlier stages of the disease. Once chronic aerocystitis has developed no treatment will be effective and such racers are better culled.

Erythromycin, tetracyclines, tylosine, tiamulin have been given with success. Injections of dihydrostreptomycin or spectinomycin are effective in individual birds. Belgian investigators have found that mycoplasma is resistent to erythromycin.

Control

To prevent re-infection following treatment or spread of the disease after possible contact, regular disinfection of water containers is recommended. The addition of a chlorine-based disinfectant to the drinking water helps to control the disease.

3. Pseudotuberculosis

Pseudotuberculosis is a sporadically-occurring disease of many species of birds, occuring very occasionally in pigeons. The disease is caused by Yersinia (Pasteurella) pseudotuberculosis and the infection in pigeons is transmitted from wild birds, rabbits or infected rodents especially rats and mice.

Symptoms

The disease affects mainly young birds and pigeons in poor condition. Diarrhoea, with severe thirst, progresses to inappetence, dehydration, emaciation, severe weakness and death. Very often only one or two pigeons in a loft of 50 or a 100 birds, are affected and it would appear as if cases are more prevalent in the warmer summer months.

Pathology

At autopsy the most striking aspect is the multitude of miliary creamy-white nodules, scattered throughout the carcase but particularly present in the abdominal organs. The liver is enlarged and the spleen, intestine and pancreas are affected. The gut may show an haemorrhagic enteritis.

Diagnosis

The similarity to other diseases with a non-specific loss of condition, precludes a diagnosis being made in the live bird and autopsy is performed. The postmortem examination is strongly suggestive, but the final diagnosis is dependant on the results of bacterial cultures. Histopathological examination may be required to exclude other possibilities.

Treatment and Control

Because of its sporadic nature, the disease is not a problem and treatment is not usually advised. Yersinia organisms are susceptible to tetracyclines and, in special cases, treatment with selected drugs may be tried.
     Control is achieved through the eradication of all rodents from the loft and preventing their access to the food containers.

4. Aspergillosis

Aspergillosis is an acute or chronic infection of birds including pigeons, predominantly affecting the respiratory system. It is characterised by typical white or grey-green plaques, growth colonies of the causative fungus, Aspergillus fumigatus on the airsacs.

Etiology

Aspergillus fumigatus is a common spore-forming organism in nature and is mainly a secondary pathogen, causing disease when resistance is already lowered by some other condition. Under ideal conditions, aspergillosis is an acute primary disease, the main etiological factor being the massive presence of infective spores in the immediate environment.
     Ideal conditions are the presence of warmth and moisture. In the colder and wetter parts of the country, many fanciers favour a

floor covering of straw in the lofts. Should the straw become wet, the fungus can rapidly multiply and lead to mammoth presence of infective spores, increasing the risk of an outbreak. Training and racing panniers, prepared with moist straw bedding, run a similar risk. The chronic disease affects individual pigeons.

Symptoms

Acute and chronic forms of the disease are clearly distinguished. The acute form occurs in young pigeons, particularly following weaning. The youngsters become apathetic, lose appetite, huddle, and lose weight. Some respiratory distress is seen and death occurs in five or six days.

The chronic form occurs in adult birds, and has a more gradual onset. An affected pigeon has often been debilitated by another condition. Treatment of the primary condition is then only partially successful. The striking feature is one of weight loss. The bird has respiratory distress seen in a round gaping epiglottis, decreased appetite, depression, loss of weight to emaciation and eventually open mouth breathing, gasping and death. With the bird held in the hand one can often discern sagging of the abdomen. Respiratory rales or gurgling is not heard.

Pathology

Autopsy examination findings of the two forms, differ markedly.

Acute form. The carcase is thin, toxic and dehydrated. On opening the abdomen a purulent, bright yellow liquid, is seen in the airsacs and lungs, which are severely affected.

Chronic form. The autopsy is very typical. In the initial stages small plaques of fungal growth is found on the lungs or in the abdominal airsacs. In a severely affected bird these grow to become large hollow cavities in the abdomen – up to two centimetres in diameter. On the exterior these cavities have a fleshy appearance, but their interior is covered with whitish or grey-green fuzzy fungal growth – similar to the growth seen on stale bread. The carcase is emaciated, dehydrated and usually shows signs of other disease processes.

Diagnosis

In a very valuable pigeon in which the disease is suspected, a laparoscopy can be performed, but the diagnosis is usually made on the typical postmortem findings. The diagnosis is confirmed by microscopical examination of the lesion, or culture of the fungus.

Treatment and Control

Treatment is not usually attempted though success has been claimed following oral administration of Mycostatin (susp. of nystatin – not absorbed from the intestine in mammals). Fogging with a standard fungicide can be tried in a valuable pigeon.

Flucytozine (Alcoban) is absorbed from the gut, excreted via the kidneys and is effective against Aspergillus 'in vitro'. It should be effective in curing chronic cases (has not been tried), but the extensive tissue proliferation and disturbance of the normal anatomy that occurs following an outbreak of the disease, prevents previously-infected race pigeons from competing successfully.

Control is important and with correct management it will not be a problem. Straw must not be used in the loft or panniers but if unavoidable, the obvious precautions should be taken. When the origin and previous storage of the straw are unknown, as when purchased from a dealer or farmer, the straw should be carefully examined. Only healthy straw should be used.

Healthy straw has a gleaming, pale yellow colour and a sweet, dry and clean smell, as if it's been freshly cut. Wet straw is thrown out. All bales known to have been exposed to moisture, are rejected, even if they appear to be in order. Any sign of mouldiness is bad and the bale thrown out. A greyish powdery discolouration of the stalks is suspicious and the whole bale is rejected. The bales are weighed and the lightest, which are most likely to be the healthiest, selected.

5. Candidiasis

Candidiasis is not a common disease of pigeons. The disease, caused by the fungus Candida albicans, usually affects the digestive tract especially the crop, and is characterised by the formation of necrotic patches with some ulceration.

Symptoms

Whitney describes loss of condition, vomiting, thickened crop walls, ulcerative patches in the mouth and "sourcrop". Delayed filling, with the crop resembling a plastic bag full of water, is an early and frequent sign.

"Sourcrop" is regularly but infrequently seen, particularly in the summer months in breeding stock. Whether the condition is always caused by an infection of Candida albicans, has yet to be established.

Pathology

On autopsy the bird has white circular lesions in the lining of the crop. The carcase is dehydrated and cachectic.

Treatment

Emptying the crop and dosing with nystatin (20 000 units/ day) (Mycostatin – 0.5 ml) gives good results. This is repeated twice daily until recovery. Amphotericin B (Fungizone), related to nystatin, is also effective. Flucytosine (Alcoban) prevents fungal multiplication and is well absorbed from the intestine (excreted via the urine).

Chapter 6

Protozoal diseases

1. Coccidiosis

Coccidiosis is a protozoal disease affecting the intestinal tract and occurring in practically all species of livestock and birds. It is well-known to pigeon fanciers across the world and many remedies, inherited mainly from poultry farming, are available for treatment of the condition. Though mortalities are generally low the disease is important to racing fanciers because of its 'erosive element'. Most adult pigeons have some resistance to coccidiosis and are coccidia carriers without showing visible signs of the disease.

Coccidiosis generally affects the health of pigeons in two ways. It damages the intestinal lining facilitating the entry of other more pathogenic organims (eg. E. coli), and/or it exacerbates the pathology caused by other bowel diseases (eg. hairworms).

Incidence

Well-known to animal keepers the world over, the disease occurs in most species and severe mortalities have occurred in dogs, sheep, cattle and particularly chickens. It occurs in many species of birds, but is typically host-specific, so that coccidiosis of pigeons do not affect any other animal or bird and vice versa. Chickens or dogs defaecating where pigeons forage, eg. on grass or in the garden, do not constitute any danger for pigeons.

Etiology

Two causative organisms, Eimeria columbarum and E.labbeana, are involved in the pathogenesis of pigeon coccidiosis. Morphologically there is little difference between them and, as no obvious pathological or clinical differences are apparent, we make no distinction between the species. To fully understand how coccidiosis affects the health of its host, we examine the lifecycle.

Lifecycle

Three stages take place in the lifecycle.

1. Asexual stage

The cycle begins with the ingestion of sporulated oocysts by the pigeon. These oocysts contain the infective sporozoites, which are released when the pigeon's intestinal system digests the oocyst wall. The released sporozoites are motile, penetrate the cells lining the digestive tract, grow to form trophozoites and continue to develop to schizonts. The nuclei of the shizonts undergo a process of division, which ends in the formation of merozoites, that closely resemble the sporozoites which first entered the cell. Having grown to a ripe stage, both the cell and the schizont rupture, releasing a flood of merozoites which, acting like sporozoites, immediately set about finding a new intestinal cell to enter. This completes the asexual cycle.

  The process, which takes place in 24 hours, is then repeated several times. A single oocyst has been calculated to be able to produce 2.5 million merozoites, destroying innumerable intestinal cells in the process.

2. Sexual stage

After a number of asexual reproductions as described above, a sexual reproductive process is begun. This involves the third-generation merozoites, which, upon entering an intestinal cell, differentiate into microgametocytes or macrogametocytes. The mobile microgametocytes, upon release, seek out the macrogame-tocytes and effect fertilization. Once this occurs, the fertilised macrogametocyte, now known as the zygote, undergoes further changes resulting into an unsporulated oocyst. Oocysts are passed in the droppings of the bird about four or five days after ingestion of the original sporulated oocyst.

3. External stage

Upon excretion of the oocyst in the faeces, a stage of sporulation, which is dependent upon heat, moisture and oxygen, begins. Under these favourable conditions the process is completed in one or two days. Unless sporulation is completed, the oocysts are not infective and cannot repeat the cycle when ingested. Sporulated oocysts are able to survive for extended periods (months or even years) under favourable conditions – such as in moist manure or water containers.

Epidemiology

Coccidiosis is spread by the dissemination of oocyst-infected droppings and contamination of the food and water. Overcrowding, poor ventilation, unhygienic feeding and watering, accumulation of faeces on the floor and in cracks and crevices, all contribute to oocyst build-up in a colony of pigeons. Under conditions of stress,

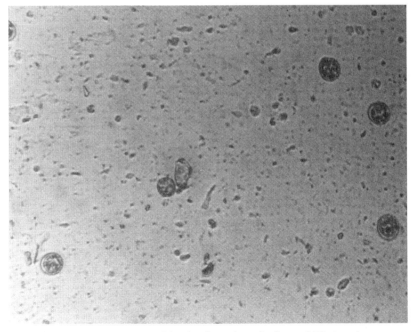

Coccidiosis, occysts as passed in the droppings (enlarged 70 times).

(eg. racing, breeding, worms, disease or malnutrition), problems with coccidiosis must be expected.

In contrast to most other animal species, pigeons do not appear

to develop an immunity to coccidiosis. However, it seems that some sort of premunity develops, as adult birds in general are more resistant to infection. Control measures as in poultry, where young chicks are allowed to build a low-grade infection to stimulate immunity, do not function as effectively in pigeons.

Pathogenesis and Symptoms

Knowing the lifecycle, it is easier to understand how coccidiosis affects the pigeon. When the schizont ruptures from the intestinal epithelium, it causes haemorrhage, inflammation and necrosis of the area. One ingested oocyst can produce 2.5 million merozoites and with the rupture of each shizont, an intestinal lining cell is destroyed. Severe infestation causes considerable damage. Depending on the degree of resistance and stress levels, variable secondary bacterial invasion takes place.

1. Acute form

This form occurs mainly in young birds and though more serious clinically, it rarely occurs. It causes an enteritis, which is easily recognisable and corrective treatment is readily implemented. The defense mechanisms of young birds at three to four weeks are not yet fully active, so babies are weaned at a most vulnerable time. Food and drink are often ignored while the young pigeons learn to look after themselves, increasing their stress level.

The intestinal epithelium is destroyed by rupturing schizonts and large sections may be lost, causing intestinal damage and diarrhoea. Once a breach has been made into the first defense line of the intestine, bacteria invade the damaged portions, causing further inflammation. Soft, slimy or watery droppings, are seen, rarely with blood. (Blood is commonly found in the droppings of chickens and other animals suffering from coccidiosis, but not in pigeons). Emaciation, dehydration, weakness, paralysis and death may follow. Death is caused by dehydration, as affected birds lose vast quantities of fluid and cease eating and drinking. Secondary bacterial invaders affect the internal organs.

Vitamin deficiencies may result as a further complication at a time that vitamins are most needed. Sick birds respond well to treatment, the bowel having remarkable powers of recuperation.

2. Subclinical Form

This form is a typical erosion disease. The birds appear to be in good health, eat normally, exercise well and their droppings may be firm and have good colour. In races, however, they do not perform well.

1. Microlesions in the intestine cause a mild disturbance, which may become chronic and hamper the proper functioning of the bowel. The carbohydrates, proteins, vitamins and minerals, essential for attaining peak condition, cannot be absorbed.

2. Bacteria entering through the microlesions invade the bloodstream, spread to various parts of the body and set up foci of infection in the liver, spleen, kidneys and other organs. These are contained by the defense mechanism of the pigeon but the process uses energy destined for conditioning the bird and the bird is thus deprived of sufficient reserves to develop peak physical fitness.

3. If peak fitness is missing, the bird cannot respond to the stresses of training and instead of building strength and resistance, the opposite occurs. The training is wasted and the bird is physically weaker than before.

4. Not being at peak fitness, the pigeon's general resistance to stressful conditions such as hard racing, is decreased and it falls prey to the other pigeon scourges like trichomoniasis, paratyphoid etc.

5. During a hard race a bird needs all its available energy but because the glucose reserves are lowered, general resistance decreases further and the mild form of coccidiosis becomes more severe, with further debilitation. A vicious cycle begins. Either the pigeon cannot finish the race, trapping into a strange loft, spreading oocysts, or it returns home, debilitated and dehydrated.

Despite good care, it takes a long time to recuperate and replenish its reserves. It might not be able to, having sometimes suffered permanent damage to heart and kidneys. Such a bird occasionally must to be destroyed, because, even though appearing to be in good physical condition, the slightest stress weakens it. Never again will it be a successful racer. Such birds are often kept, only to be lost on the first race subsequent to their recuperation. They are, however, capable of breeding good offspring.

Diagnosis

The acutely-ill pigeon with diarrhoea, is readily diagnosed as suffering from coccidiosis and the diagnosis is confirmed micro-scopically, with many oocysts seen in a fresh faeces sample.

A subclinical case presents more difficulty. Bearing in mind that some oocysts are likely to be found in the excreta of all pigeons under average good hygienic conditions, we have adopted a quantitative method that has given satisfactory results over a number of years.

Procedure

The dropping from a suspected bird is placed on a glass slide and the white urate deposits are carefully removed. (This is helpful as the urate crystals hinder examination by masking the presence of oocysts). The pasty faeces is mixed with a small amount of water – enough to make a liquid suspension – and spread thinly and evenly over the surface of the slide. Examination under a medium lens (100 X magnification) reflects a realistic picture of the degree of infection. If, on average, more than four oocysts are discovered per field, treatment is recommended.

At least 5 to 10% of birds are examined from each loft, ensuring that a representative sample is obtained. Very often two birds out of five examined will be negative, whereas the other three are positive. The degree of infection of the worst case is used to evaluate the status of infection in the loft and to decide whether treatment is necessary.

Severe infections may be found in lofts that were treated only a few days before. The situation arises either from inadequate treatment, which includes drug resistance, or more commonly, from reinfection. Obtaining a history of treatments given, is essential. We will return to this later.

Treatment

Because of the widespread nature of the disease, innumerable articles and papers have been written about the treatment and prevention in other species. Many medications have been advocated over the years. Pigeon fanciers gained in a spin-off from poultry research, as most drugs developed and used in poultry against coccidiosis, are used with success in pigeons. Most of these medications belong to the sulphonamides and though potentially harmful in overdosage, they have served the fancy well. Some of the more common are: sulphaquinoxaline (Embazin), sulphadimidine, (Sulfazine), sulphachlorapyrazine (Esb 3, Coxytrol) and amprolium (Amprol).

In recent years other medications, like clazuril (Appertex) and toltrazuril (Baycox), have been developed.

Following a course of treatment, I have found it advantageous to administer the B-group vitamins.

Treatment with antibiotics may appear to effect a cure in some cases, but this is owing to their effect on the secondary invaders. I particularly like sulphamezathine, because it has a beneficial effect against coccidia, as well as secondary invaders.

Control

Absolute hygiene is the only way of keeping coccidiosis out of a loft. The cleaner the loft, the better and it must be dry at all times. Water spillages must be mopped up as soon as possible.

The loft must be meticulously clean, which means that no excreta is allowed to accumulate in the loft, neither under the perches nor in the feeding area. The pigeons are preferably fed in a trough that is sealed when not in use. Even if the birds are not fed on the floor, coccidia tend to accumulate there and pigeons ingest oocysts by pecking at any interesting object.

The floor must be smooth, without cracks or crevices. A wooden plank floor with joins (tongue and groove) that are slightly open, is not good enough. Such a floor must be overlaid with an impervious smooth lining such as tempered hardboard, plywood sheeting etc.

The introduction of new birds into a loft is carefully monitored. Extra care should be employed when birds are basketed together for races, particularly if water is supplied. One infected pigeon soiling the water trough, can be responsible for spreading coccidiosis into the loft of every member of that club. Should such equipment not be disinfected and cleaned regularly, it can remain a source of infection for the duration of the racing season.

Pigeons that are kept stress-free under hygienic conditions, have been known to remain coccidia-free for months and in this way have sidestepped a major obstacle to becoming successful racers.

2. Trichomoniasis (Crop canker)

Trichomoniasis is an infectious protozoal disease of many species of birds with a special prevalence for doves and pigeons. It is caused by a unicellular flagellate, Trichomonas columbae, has a worldwide distribution and is familiar to all fanciers who have been in the sport for some time. Significant in the racing of pigeons, it presents as an acute disease with a high mortality

amongst younger stock or as an erosion disease with a chronic
course, in older racers.

Etiology

Crop canker is caused by an infection with Trichomonas columbae,
a motile protozoal organism with four flagellae at the anterior end,
which give the organism motility and enhance its microscopic visi-
bility. The parasites occur in and is pathogenic to many animal
species, in particular the doves, falcons and hawks. (Raptors
become infected after feeding on infected pigeons and doves).
Other relatives of the parasite are found naturally in many species
of birds (ducks, turkeys, owls, hawks, grouse, coots, cormorants
etc.), without apparent harm to the host. Pathogenic species e.g. T.
foetus and T. vaginalis inhabit the genital tract of bovine and
primate species and can be difficult to eradicate.

    According to Whitney, five strains of the parasite have been
identified in pigeons, with three occurring to any great extent. We
see three distinct forms of the disease but whether these are
caused by different individual strains, has yet to be determined.

Epidemiology

It appears as if pigeons are natural hosts to trichomonas with
almost every pigeon hosting the organism in the crop and gullet.
Premunity exists in adult birds but its duration and effectiveness
is stress-related.

    Transmission of the disease occurs when pigeons are billing and
feeding young. It has been demonstrated by Stabler that newly-
hatched squabs are infected at their first feed. Drinking from a
communal water bowl spreads the infection between adult birds in
the loft.

    The disease is more prevalent during the summer months and
we see a marked reduction in the incidence of acute cases in
winter. This is probably related to better survival of the organism
outside the body of its host when outside temperatures are closer
to normal body temperature. At temperatures of 25°C and above,
moist grains have maintained viable

    T. gallinae for at least 13 days. Trichomonas will survive for one
whole day in water at 25°C.

Clinical Signs and Pathogenesis

Signs of infection appear a week after introduction of the

organism. One of three forms can occur.

1. Classical (acute) form.

This form of the disease usually occurs in youngsters, from babies in the nest until two to three months after weaning. The birds are obviously sick, with ruffled feathers, loose watery droppings, loss of weight, excessive thirst and decreased appetite. They are apathetic, lose interest in their surroundings and may be picked up without moving. When this stage is reached mortalities must be expected. Such babies probably would never have developed into strong racers should they have survived and it is better to cull them at this stage.

Symptoms

Upon examination the bird will usually have yellow cheesy growths in the throat, adherent to the mucosa. Many stages of severity occur. We see one or two match-head size lesions, indicating a more resistant bird to one with large cheesy lumps, nearly filling the throat and mouth and hindering eating. The growths may encroach upon the epiglottis, causing respiratory distress. From the throat, infection may spill over into the upper airways and spread to the internal organs, especially the liver and heart.

A less prevalent form occurs in nestlings where the navel is affected. Infection spreads rapidly from the enlarged navel area to the abdomen and the liver. The abdomen appears pendulous, swollen and soft and the baby rapidly loses weight and dies. Severe liver damage occurs and though treatment might save the life, a healthy robust bird cannot be produced; culling is preferable.

2. Obstructive form

I have categorised this form only because the predilection site of the parasite leads to a distinct disease syndrome. It is probably caused by a singular strain of T. columbae, not occurring commonly. The morbidity in a flock is high, in the region of 60 to 70%, with a 100% mortality.

Symptoms

Birds of all ages are affected, even though they are initially in good condition and the occurrence of outbreaks is not related to stress levels. Initially, the pigeons appear to eat and drink normally but gradually lose condition. Some birds may vomit. At a more advanced stage, the pigeons are unable to swallow their food, stand very upright with heads high, necks stretched and make repeated efforts at swallowing. Their crops are full of water but the pigeons gradually become more and more dehydrated, lose weight and die. Numerous trichomonads are seen on microscopic examination of a throat swab.

Autopsy

The typical yellow caseous lesions of trichomoniasis are found in the short area of the distal oesophagus, between the crop and the proventriculus. This section lies in the thoracic inlet, which is narrow and serves as entrance for the gullet and trachea to the inside of the body. The organisms attack the oesphageal epithelium here and produce the typical cheesy growths which enlarge, invade the surrounding tissues and occlude the thoracic inlet. Total obstruction to the passage of food and water follows, with starvation, dehydration and death.

Usually no other signs of trichomoniasis are seen. In a few cases the pressure is more severe on the trachea causing marked respiratory distress with a drooping tail, heaving sternum and open-mouth breathing. Death quickly ensues.

The invasive yellow growths have been seen in the throat and mouth area (palate, side of mouth etc) and causing the deaths of large numbers of free-living wild doves, since 1991. It is a highly contagious, fatal infection and its locality is very specific, occurring nowhere else in the body. More recently (1992) the infection has appeared in adult racing pigeons but in sporadic instances. It is thought that a specific strain is responsible for the symptoms.

3. Subclinical form

All the birds that are carriers of trichomonads and are not showing signs of the disease, are grouped here. They have had the disease and recovered, or may never have shown a sign of ill health. (It is contentious whether they ought to be known as carriers of the infection or as birds with a premunity. They are not carriers in the sense that we normally understand the term.)

I do not believe that a truly symbiotic relationship can exist between a racing pigeon and trichomonad parasites. For a pigeon to be able to perform regularly at its best, it must have no parasites. Health alone is not sufficient – it must possess super health.

Any evidence of meaningful numbers of trichomonads found in the throat of a pigeon involved in racing, is detrimental to its chances of being successful.

Within the concept of subclinical infection many stages are seen.

The most severe usually have one or two yellow lesions in the back of the throat, but show no sign of ill-health. Others may demonstrate numerous white spots, pinhead in size, on the curtain in the back of the throat. These spots are of no consequence at this stage as they are healed, calcified lesions of a previous attack of canker. (There is still some doubt as to the etiology of these spots; Signs of herpesvirus infection, abscesses caused by E. coli, calcoliths in the salivary glands etc., have all been popular as causes.) The spots are seen most often in yearling pigeons and generally disappear after a few months. They do not respond to treatment and do not interfere with racing – if the bird no longer has active trichomoniasis.

Some birds have lost a section of the curtain from a previous episode of crop canker. This will not affect their racing provided there are no active trichomonads.

The largest group of birds are those that have never shown any obvious sign of infection, yet upon microscopic examination are found to harbour many organisms. These are the carriers, regarded as healthy by many fanciers but who consist of the real problem, by reducing the performance of a race team and being a constant source of weak and sickly babies in a breeding loft. At best they reproduce the carrier state in their offspring, who perpetuate their poor racing performance. Any 'better' breeding stock, introduced from another loft, is soon reduced to the standard of the old stock, as infection spreads and their offspring suffer the same fate as that of their predecessors.

Virulence and Immunity.

At present there is no explanation for the divergence of virulence, seen in the various strains of T. columbae. Neither are there satisfactory explanations for the mechanism of immunity to the infection or the mechanisms which reduce that immunity and produce the typical lesions.

We know that:

1. Various strains, varying in virulence, exist.

2. Cross-immunity exists between virulent and avirulent strains.

3. When a bird has been immunised by exposure and survives, it retains its immunity for over one year.

4. When immune birds are subjected to challenge by a virulent strain they can become carriers of the virulent strain and transmit it to other birds.

I have gone into some detail above, so that the reader may understand why it is desirable that every racing bird is treated. Because immunity exists in exposed, recovered birds, they can become carriers of a virulent strain. If at some stage, owing to stress factors of racing or breeding, the immunity breaks down, these birds would be susceptible immediately to the virulent strain, which they are carrying with them. At any time they are able to pass this virulent strain to a non-immune loftmate or to their own progeny.

Trichomoniasis is ubiquitous and I believe that breeding stock need not be kept sterile of the germ but be allowed to build up a mild trichomonad population. Continued careful monitoring and treatment at the first sign of disease, allows youngsters to build some immunity before they are transferred to the main loft. In the race loft, particularly during the racing season, all birds must be sterile of trichomonads as far as possible.

Diagnosis.

The obviously sick acutely-affected youngster with yellow growths choking his throat, is practically self-diagnostic. Confirmation is obtained by squashing a little of the inspissated pus, mixing it with a few drops of water on a glass slide and microscopically demonstrating thousands of trichomonads. Internal forms of trichomoniasis can only be diagnosed on autopsy.

The subclinical form is easily demonstrated. A cotton bud is moistened and a throat and crop swab is taken. (If a cotton bud is too short to reach into the crop, a home-made swab , made from a splintered tongue depressor and cotton wool, serves equally well.) With an assistant holding the pigeon, the examiner holds the bird's head, stretches the neck and opens the mouth with one hand. With the other hand he introduces the cotton bud into the pigeon's throat and down into the crop, where it is moved up and down five or six times, in order to collect mucus. The cotton is now squeezed out over a glass slide and a drop of the liquid is examined under a microscope at medium (100 X) magnification.

Once warmed by the microscope light source, the trichomonads appear mobile and jiggle together in small clumped groups, or if in single state, they move briskly in small haphazard circles or spin dizzily. It is essential that at least 5-10% of the birds per loft are examined, because it not infrequently happens that two or three birds are negative with the fourth and fifth strongly positive. Only one strongly positive bird out of five examined, is needed to recommend treatment for the whole group. Re-examination, two weeks following treatment is strongly recommended.

Differential Diagnosis.

Crop canker must be distinguished from two other disease conditions:

1. Diphtheroid pox

Position. The yellow pox lesions in the mouth and throat may resemble crop canker but the lesions of pox, resulting when birds have fought, are usually more in the front, middle and side of the mouth. Canker is seen further back in the throat.

Adhesiveness. Pox lesions are well attached to the underlying mucosa and have a good blood supply, bleeding profusely if forcibly removed, whereas canker growths are fairly loose and do not bleed much if removed.

Other signs. The pigeon with diptheroid pox, or its loftmates, will usually have external pox lesions.

Microscopical. The pigeon with pox may test negatively for the presence of trichomonads, the canker bird will always be positive. Be aware that some birds have both pox and cropcanker.

2. Pigeonherpes virus (PHV)

Differentiation from cropcanker may be difficult, especially where both conditions occur together.
Pathogenicity. PHV is the more pathogenic condition. Affected birds are extremely dull and listless and appear to be sleepy, oblivious to their environment.

Adhesiveness. PHV does not cause distinct lumps of pus, but tends to coat the mouth and throat with a purulent exudate which is non-adherent to the mucosa. Lesions of PHV emit a rotten stench.

Response to treatment. Birds affected by PHV do not respond to treatment.

Confirmation. Virus isolation is the only method of confirming an herpesvirus outbreak. Finding intranulear inclusions in the liver is strongly suggestive.

Treatment

Flock treatment

Spin-offs from the pig and poultry industies gave us first 2-amino-5-nitrothiazole (Enheptin, Entramin, tricoxine etc.), and later dimetridazole (Emtryl, Dovatric etc.). Metronidazole (Flagyl, Meditrich), carnidazole (Spartrix) and ronidazole (Ridsol S, Tricho-plus) are now added to the list and have a wide spectrum of safety. All the remedies are excellent and can be used with success, but in all cases control checks must be done two weeks later to test effi-cacy of treatment.

See chapter 18 for the correct application and dosages of the mentioned products. Vitamin/mineral preparations are strongly recommended after any course of specific treatment.

Individual treatment

Single valuable pigeons can be treated by first gently removing as many lesions from the mouth and throat as possible, after which a concentrated solution of dimetridazole (Emtryl) or 2% iodine solu-tion is brushed onto the affected parts. Metronidazole, in pill form, may be given instead of the dimetridazole and an antibiotic injec-tion is always included to treat secondary infections.

Control

Control of the disease and prevention of acute outbreaks must revolve around:

1. Regular treatment.

2. No breeding during high summer.

3. Careful attention to hygiene – especially regarding regular disinfection of water troughs, clean fresh water and never allowing food to become soiled.

4. Careful surveillance of the number of pigeons kept per unit of loft space. Overcrowding, especially in summer, can lead to explosive outbreaks of the disease. (Maximum number is two pigeons per cubic metre.)

3. Malaria

Malaria of pigeons is an infectious disease caused by protozoa of the genus Plasmodium and transmitted by infected mosquitoes of the genera Culex, Aedes and Anopheles. The disease has not been recorded in temperate countries, as far as we are aware.

The similarity of symptoms and difficulty of differentiation on blood slides from an infection of Haemoproteus spp, has resulted in the latter being loosely referred to as malaria. This is false and I believe that the two diseases should be recognised and dealt with independently. To maintain the distinction we have given the name pseudomalaria to an infection with Haemoproteus.

Etiology and Transmission

About 50 different species of avian malarial parasites have been described. Of these Plasmodium relictum and Plasmodium matutinum, are responsible for malaria in pigeons and doves. They are biologically transmitted by mosquitoes only.

Symptoms

Severe infections cause anaemia, droopiness and loss of condition, decreased endurance and birds flying with open beaks. Susceptibility to other disease conditions is increased and birds will have trichomoniasis, coccidiosis and mycoplasmosis.

Pathology

Severe cases will have an anaemic carcase, swollen, dark-coloured, almost black spleen, pale, swollen kidneys and loss of condition.

Diagnosis

Microscopic examinations of stained bloodslides reveal the presence of plasmodium (shizonts or trophozoites) in the cytoplasm of the erythrocytes. The trophozoites of plasmodium are small, irregularly shaped bodies, while the shizonts are larger and may push the nucleus of the erythrocyte to one side.

Treatment and Control

According to Keymer most of the human anti-malarial drugs should be effective. Quinacrine (mepacrine) hydrochloride has been sucessfully used against malaria in canaries.

4. Pseudomalaria

The name was coined for a malaria-like disease caused by an infection with Haemoproteus spp. and serves to distinguish the disease from true malaria, caused by Plasmodium spp. The two diseases are discussed separately.

Etiology and Transmission

Haemoproteus columbae and H. sacharovi transmitted by the pigeon fly (louse fly), Pseudolynchia canariensis (syn. maura) and the midge Culicoides, are the cause of pseudomalaria in pigeons. Pseudomalaria is not transmitted by mosquitoes. According to Cook, other insects may also be involved in transmitting the parasites but the possibility has not yet been sufficiently investigated.

Symptoms

Pigeon malaria is a more important factor in pigeon racing than what is generally realised. This is so because, with the exception of the extreme cases, affected pigeons show no clinical signs of ill-health, yet these birds are incapable of performing as well as their breeding allows.

Mildly infected pigeons show no abnormalities. They appear so well as to occasionally lead to the assumption that they are in top form. Many of the signs of fitness are present, feathering is smooth, musculature is full and supple and good birds are sent to difficult races. But they fail to perform. On a hard race, infected birds lag behind and some do not return.

Moderately infected pigeons show no overt sign of disease but observant fanciers notice dullness and lack of form. Eating and breeding are not affected, training is subdued.

Severe infections cause anaemia, droopiness and loss of condition. Anaemia is seen in the mucous membranes of the mouth and the iris. Respiration becomes laboured. General resistance to

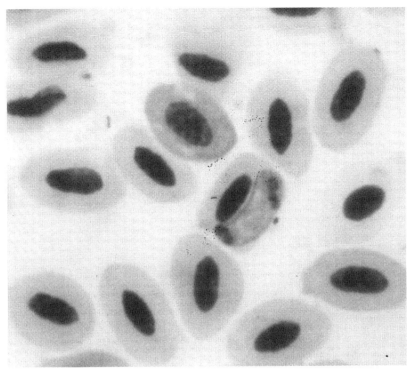

Pseudomalaria, Haemoproteus Columbae. The parasite invades the cytoplasm of the red blood cell and does not disturb the nucleus.

disease is decreased and most of the birds develop trichomoniasis, coccidiosis or mycoplasmosis.

Whereever pigeon flies are not strictly controlled, the disease is prevalent and infection rates of 80-100% have been found. It would appear that Haemoproteus is more prevalent than Plasmodium and consequently of more importance, even though true malaria is more pathogenic.

Pathology

Birds killed for post mortem examination reveal few pathological changes. In a moderately infected bird, one might see a paling and slight swelling of the kidneys. This is not a constant finding. Severe cases show an anaemic carcase, swollen dark-coloured almost black spleen, pale swollen kidneys and loss of condition. The spleen is often 5 or 6 times the size of the normal.

Diagnosis

Microscopic examinations of stained bloodslides reveal the presence of Haemoproteus (gametocytes only) in the cytoplasm of erythrocytes. Haemoproteus typically has a halter appearance with both ends of the parasite folding around the nucleus of the red blood cell without displacement of the nucleus. The trophozoites of Plasmodium, from which they must be differentiated, are smaller irregularly shaped bodies, while the shizonts are larger and push the nucleus of the erythrocyte to one side.

Treatment and Control

According to Keymer, most of the human anti-malarial drugs are effective. We have found that treatment must be continued for some days with constant monitoring of the blood. It appears as if the parasites are more resistant to treatment in some birds than in others. Treatment with primaquin sulphate (Antemal) has given us excellent results.

   Control consists of keeping the loft free of pigeon flies, the chief vectors. Spraying the loft once a year with an effective contact insecticide (eg. permethrins – Coopex, Ambush), will do this adequately. See chapter 19 for more details of this procedure.

5. Hexamitiasis

Hexamitiasis causes catarrhal enteritis in turkeys, pigeons and some other birds. Hexamita columbae is the causal organism in pigeons. It is a microscopic organism, smaller than Trichomonas, with two nuclei and eight flagellae and is extremely motile. The parasite is strongly host-specific for pigeons.

Symptoms

Profuse watery diarrhoea is the striking feature of the disease. The birds sit huddled up, become anorexic, dehydrated and lose weight. Parasites occur throughout the length of the intestine and must be differentiated from Giardia and Trichomonas. They are smaller than Trichomonas and move more rapidly in a linear fashion.

Diagnosis

The diagnosis is established by microscopically demonstrating the organisms in fresh faeces. Old faeces will not show the organism.

Treatment

Hexamitiasis is successfully treated with dimetridazole (Emtryl, Dovatric etc.) + furazolidone (or another chemotherapeutic) for five days.

6. Toxoplasmosis

Toxoplasmosis has a worldwide distribution and is best known as a serious disease of humans, particularly children. Many species of animals can be infected but few reliable records in pigeons exist. Finlay & Manwell stated that in some areas the incidence of toxoplasmosis is high, and the disease has been isolated from pigeons on sporadic occasions.

Symptoms

As a group, birds frequently harbour the organisms with no clinical evidence of disease. Symptoms when they occur are variable. Whitney cited shortness of breath, diarrhoea, loss of weight and anaemia. Chickens show anorexia, emaciation, paleness, diarrhoea and blindness and one could expect these symptoms to occur in pigeons.

Diagnosis

The diagnosis can be made on laboratory tests only; either by demonstrating antibodies to the toxoplasms or by culture of the specimens. Autopsy reveals pneumonia, pleuritis and various other disease patterns and even some negative results. More research is necessary to determine the distribution and importance of the disease in racing pigeons.

Control

Because the toxoplasm organisms are ubiquitous and so little is known about their transmission, the general principles of disease prevention are followed. The more important of these are avoidance of overcrowding, maintenance of good sanitation, and performance of autopsies on all dead birds.

6. Leucocytozoonosis

Seventeen species of doves and pigeons have been found to be
infected with Leucocytozoon marchouxi, which is found only in
birds. In South Africa the parasite was found in domestic pigeons
by Jansen. With a disease common in birds and a life history
similar to plasmodium and haemoproteus, it would seem that the
disease might become widely spread in our country. In the USA
the disease is as commonly found as haemoproteus.

As yet little is known of the clinical signs and pathogenesis of
leucocytozoonosis in pigeons. Transmission is by Simulium (black
fly) and Culicoides midges.

Diagnosis

Diagnosis is made by demonstrating the organisms in the cytoplasm of the leucocytes (and sometimes in the erythrocytes), where
they take over almost all of the cell, pushing the nucleus to one
side and distorting the cell.

Transmission

The blackfly (Simulium spp) is the reported vector for leucocytozoonosis in birds and probably is for pigeons, also.

Control and Treatment

If the blackfly is the vector, as assumed, control of the disease
would centre around control of the fly.

No treatment is recorded but it is suggested that quinacrine may
be effective against the mature stages.

Chapter 7

Parasitic diseases

A. ENDOPARASITES (Internal worms)

More has been said and written about worm maladies and remedies than about possibly any other form of disease occurring in pigeons and, while usually under control, verminosis is a constant threat to the health and well-being of pigeons.

The problem may be divided into two main categories. All the worm types have either a direct lifecycle, which means that the worm does not require an intermediate host to complete its lifecycle, or an indirect lifecycle where some other form of life fulfils the role of intermediate host.

Those with a direct lifecycle :
        1. Ascarids.........Ascaridia columbae.
        2. Strongyles.......Ornithostrongylus quadriradiatus.
        3. Hairworms........Capillaria species.

Those with an indirect lifecycle :
        1. Tapeworms........All cestodes.
        2. Flukes...........All trematodes.
        3. Proventricular worms – Acuaria spiralis, Tetrameres spp.
        4. Gapeworms.
        5. Eyeworms.

The lifecycle is the series of processes that an organism must go through in its progression from one adult generation to the next. Antiparasitic measures attack the lifecycle, in an attempt to disrupt the series at its most vulnerable stage. It is incumbent upon the pigeon keeper to assist the wormer (vermicide) by further disruption of the lifecycle.

The lifecycle must be broken if the birds are to be kept free of internal parasites. There would be no advantage if the best medicines are used to clear the pigeons, but they are subsequently allowed to become re-infested. In no time the next outbreak would require treatment.

The more common antiparasitic drugs attack the adult stages of the worms although the better drugs are effective against additional stages. The fancier has the task of removing the pigeon droppings containing worm eggs as often as possible, (direct lifecycle) and of preventing the ingestion of infected intermediate hosts, by confinement of the pigeons to a clean area or by destruction of the intermediate host (indirect lifecycle).

Worms in pigeons are found mainly in the proventriculus (glandular stomach), small intestine and trachea. We may group them according to these localities.

1. Proventricular Worms.

1.1. ACUARIA SPIRALIS (syn. Dispharynx nasuta).
(spiral stomach worm)

This parasite occurs sporadically in pigeons and is found in the glandular stomach or proventriculus, where it causes severe damage. It has been encountered more and more frequently in recent years and is becoming a serious problem in certain countries. We have known of whole lofts wiped out through becoming infected with spiral stomach worms. The adult worms are approximately 7 to 10 mm long and burrow with their heads into the wall of the proventriculus, causing extreme irritation and damage.

Epidemiology and Lifecycle

The spiral stomach worm has an indirect lifecycle. Embryonated eggs are produced by the mature worms, pass through the digestive tract of the pigeon and are excreted in the faeces. The eggs are eaten by the common isopod crustaceans known as woodlice. (In the USA they are known as sow bugs or pill bugs). Larvae develop from the eggs, invade the tissues of the intermediate host and within one month go through two stages to become infective. No further development occurs until the intermediate host is swallowed by a pigeon.

When swallowed, the third-stage larvae are released from the crustacean tissues and move to the proventriculus (and occasionally to the oesophagus) where they attach, grow to maturity and start laying eggs. The full cycle takes about seven to eight weeks.

Some pigeons will avidly eat woodlice. The crustaceans are found in dark crevices, under stones, slabs, boards or sacking and also deep in tall grass and amongst the roots of kikuyu or other grasses. They hide from and shun direct sunlight, but pigeons manage to find them. All pill bugs and some sow bugs roll into a ball when disturbed, facilitating their uptake by pigeons.

Pathogenesis

The parasites burrow their heads into the wall of the proventriculus, eliciting an extreme proliferative reacton. Disease results through destruction of the digestive glands, excessive epithelial reaction with mechanical interference of function and toxin secretion by the worms, causing bone marrow depression and anaemia.

Symptoms

In the early stages no symptoms will be noted though the birds do not perform well. Returns from races are poor, exercise tolerance is decreased and race results become dismal. In the more advanced stages the birds lose weight, will not circle, become anaemic and the normal pasty consistency of the droppings becomes coarse as digestion becomes increasingly impaired. The epiglottis is wide open and respiratory distress is evident.

In the final stages of the disease the pigeon becomes severely anaemic as evidenced by a pale tongue and throat with loss of colour in the iris. Respiratory distress is pronounced and the abdomen feels soft, baggy and full. The breast muscles are wasted away, the pigeon is weak, barely able to fly and sits hunched up with ruffled plumage, eating a little but not digesting its food. The droppings at this stage are loose and green.

Autopsy and Diagnosis

The hugely enlarged proventriculus (up to 4x normal size), is immediately apparent and when opened reveals a medusa-like mucosa with numerous worms attached to the thickened, inflamed and slimy proventricular lining. The worms are curled up and buried beneath the slime and oedematous surface, beneath which their heads are firmly attached to the mucosa. Severe anaemia is apparent throughout the carcase. The spleen is enlarged and the intestine is inflamed with thickened, pale walls.

Histopathology of a severe case shows a myxomatosis-like acellular proventriculitis with marked vesicular congestion. There is epithelial desquamation, papillary proliferation, hypersecretion of mucus, congestion and secondary bacterial invasion of the superficial mucosa.

Diagnosis in the live bird is made by identifying the worm eggs in the faeces. A direct smear examination is adequate.

Treatment

No cure has been reported in the literature but trials with fenbendazole have shown it to be effective. Two or three doses given separately at intervals of one week were satisfactory. However we found it to be toxic at the required levels and extreme care must be taken with the dosage.

Two % diluted ivermectin solution was found effective and relatively safe for pigeons. Overdosage leads to temporary blindness in some cases, lasting about six hours, but otherwise the drug is well tolerated.

Control

Pigeons are not allowed access to grassed areas and all areas where isopods can hide must be cordoned off. The most satisfactory means of control is to keep the pigeons in the loft at all times when they are not training.

Open pens with sandy floors housing breeding birds, readily become inhabited by woodlice. At no time should crustaceans be allowed suitable living areas within reach of pigeons.

1.2. TETRAMERES AMERICANA (red stomach worm)

Marked sexual dimorphism exists, the male being extremely small and slender and the female almost spherical in shape and blood-red in colour. The female is embedded in the wall of the proventriculus and is clearly visible from the outside of the organ while the male is found free in the proventriculus or temporarily in a gland within the proventricular wall, whither it follows the female for mating.

The parasite is found with increasing regularity and its worldwide distribution appears to be spreading. Initially the effects are minimal, with only heavily parasitized birds showing symptoms, resulting in the masking of infection until the parasites have become firmly established. Having the same intermediate host, T.americana is often found with A. spiralis in the same bird or in birds from the same loft.

Lifecycle and Pathogenesis.

The life-cycle is indirect, with woodlice acting as the intermediate hosts. Embryonated eggs of the worms pass out with the faeces, are eaten by the intermediate hosts and develop to third-stage larvae, which are infective. No further development occurs until

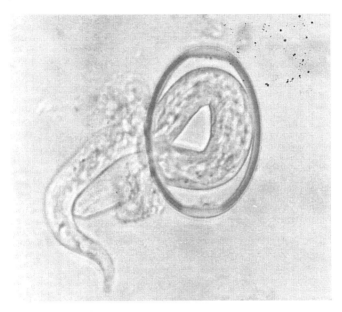

Tetrameres Americana egg, slightly squashed causing rupture of the egg and release of the larva (enlarged 400 times).

the intermediate host is swallowed by the pigeon, at which time the larvae migrate to the proventricular glands where they develop to maturity. As each female worm invades only one gland, symptoms are seen only with severe infestation. The males do not appear to cause any irritation or disease.

Symptoms

Even heavily infested birds do not appear ill but lose condition, have a lowered exercise tolerance and perform poorly in the races. Losses are heavy. The droppings lose their fine pasty consistency and appear more coarse than normal. The pectoral muscles lose suppleness, and usually feel hard, sometimes soft and flabby.

Autopsy and Diagnosis

Red stomach worms rarely cause mortality. At autopsy the proventriculus is three times the normal size, with dark-red blotches approximately 3mm by 3mm in the wall of the organ. The female worms can be popped out of the glands on the mucosal surface by applying gentle pressure around them. A deep scraping of the mucus membrane examined microscopically usually reveals the filiform male worms.

The breast muscles are atrophied and hard and the spleen is enlarged.

Diagnosis in the live bird is made by finding the typical embryonated eggs in the droppings. A direct smear sample is preferable as a saturated sugar/salt solution does not flotate the eggs and the diagnosis can be missed. A saturated zinc chloride solution crenates the eggs which alters their morphology and does not float all the eggs creating a false impression of the degree of infestation. At autopsy, demonstration of the worms is easy and conclusive.

Treatment and Control

Up to 1983, no effective treatment was available. Injectable Ivermectin was released around this time and found to be very effective for the treatment of the red stomach worm. Two injections, given one week apart gives excellent results and has proven to be relatively non-toxic at the required dosage. Overdosage causes temporary blindness.

Control is aimed at eradication of the intermediate hosts and restricting the pigeons to the loft, which must be insect-free. Bathing of the pigeons in a grassed area is not allowed. If no other suitable site is available the bath is placed either on the landing area, inside the loft or in an aviary with a concrete floor.

1.3. TETRAMERES FISSISPINA

First seen by the author in 1983, Tetrameres fissispina is rare in pigeons. It is not a normal parasite of the pigeon and herein lies its greatest threat. In repeated faeces examinations no eggs were seen in the droppings from birds later found to be infested with the

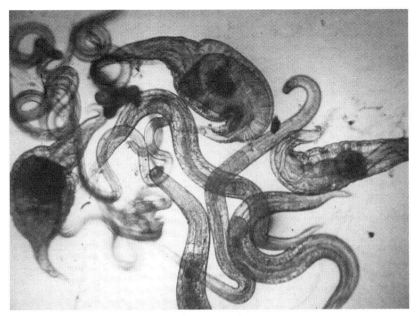

Tetrameres Fissispana (enlarged 120 times).

parasite. Microscopic examination of the female worms failed to reveal signs of egg-production. It has been postulated that because the worm finds itself in an abnormal host, no eggs are produced. This precludes the possibility of diagnosing T. fissispina in the live pigeon. Autopsy establishes the presence of the parasite but the degree of infestation is estimated from the symptoms of the remaining birds. Treatment must be on an empirical basis. T. fissispina has been found together with T. americana, suggesting that the same intermediate host is involved in the transmission of both parasites.

Symptoms

The parasite is more pathogenic than T. americana. Mildly affected birds lose condition, fly and train poorly and lose form. Severely affected birds lose appetite, become dull, dehydrated, and die.

Autopsy.

Post mortem examination reveals loss of weight to cachexia and an enlarged proventriculus. Pinpoint spots are seen, both on the external serosa and the internal mucosa. Pressure allied to the digestive glands in the wall of the organ causes the worms to pop out onto the mucosal surface.

Treatment

As the diagnosis of T. fissispina cannot be made on the live bird, evaluation of the efficacy of treatment in suspected cases, is difficult. Blanket treatment with injectable Ivermectin in lofts where the presence of the parasite had been established, resulted in a marked improvement in condition and performance of the birds.

2. Intestinal Worms

2.1. ASCARIDIA COLUMBAE (Large roundworm)

Well-known by most fanciers this worm is occasionally seen in the droppings following routine deworming programmes. It is the only ascarid worm that occurs in pigeons.

Lifecycle

The lifecycle is direct. The adult worm lays numerous eggs which are passed out in the faeces and, depending on heat and moisture, undergo a maturation process of at least two weeks. Upon completion of this process the eggs become infective and if swallowed in contaminated food or water they will excyst, releasing immature larvae into the bowel. These penetrate the mucuous membrane lining of the gut and remain there for approximately 10 to 14 days, after which they re-enter the lumen of the intestine. Eggs appear in the faeces of the pigeon, 37 to 42 days after infection.

Note 1 – During the period that the immature worms are inside the wall of the intestine they are protected from the action of local anthelmintic drugs.

Note 2 – Of the 40 days required to complete the lifecycle approximately 30 to 35 days are needed for the eggs to develop to adult worms. There is thus insufficient time for worm eggs to excyst, grow to maturity and the adult worms to begin laying eggs, before a squeaker is weaned. Consequently squeakers are weaned apparently healthy and their faeces are negative for worm eggs, even though the young birds can have massive numbers of immature worms, which develop and cause disease within two to three weeks.

Epidemiology

In warm countries many pigeon fanciers house their stock birds in a loft with a sand floor or with a sand floor aviary. The pigeons peck in the sand exposing themselves to worm infestation, because at some time, a roundworm carrier will be introduced into the loft and all the birds become infested – not necesarily becoming ill, as adult pigeons are fairly resistant to roundworms – but infesting their babies, who grow up well, but deteriorate soon after weaning.

A heavy infestation can cause severe loss of condition especially if the breeding pair is stressed by rearing rapidly-growing babies.

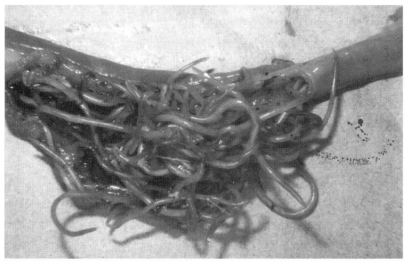

Unusually severe infestation of Ascaridia Columbae in a young bird.

A pair of healthy well-fed pigeons should be able to rear three or four rounds with two in the nest quite successfully, with no deterioration in quality of the youngsters, yet many fanciers prefer one baby to a nest. This is mainly due to incorrect feeding and internal worms.

Pathogenesis

The worms live off the food, vitamins and minerals intended for the pigeon's sustenance. They irritate the bowel mucosa mechanically and also by the production of toxic waste products. The severity of the damage they cause, is directly proportional to the numbers present.

Severe infestation in young birds can cause obstruction of the gut. Aberrant migration to and through the liver causes severe liver damage, infection and death.

Symptoms

Loss of condition occurs in all pigeons. Young birds are more severely affected and deaths may happen. Vomiting occurs and blood is occasionally present in the droppings. Adult birds are more resistant but susceptibility to other disease processes is increased. Mild infestation is reflected in lack of condition and poor race results.

Treatment and Control

The various salts of piperazine have been used for a long time and are effective but the drug has two disadvantages. A second dose is required 10 to 14 days after the first to eliminate the new generation of ascarids (see the lifecycle) and piperazine is a narrow-spectrum anthelmintic not effective against hairworms.

Products containing levamisole, pyrantel, fenbendazole, febantel, cambendazole and ivermectin can be used but side-effects must be carefully watched for. We use levamisole on a routine basis against roundworms.

Regular dosing and scrupulous hygiene will keep worm numbers under control. Eradication is extremely difficult, but a worm-free team of birds kept under ideal conditions remains clear, provided no carriers are introduced.

2.2. ORNITHOSTRONGYLUS QUADRIRADIATUS
   (Strongyle worm)

Strongyle worms occur in the crop, proventriculus and small intestine. They vary from about 1-2 cm in length, fresh worms being a reddish colour. The lifecycle is direct but shorter than that of the ascarids, and the process may be completed in 10 to 12 days under favourable circumstances. Strongyles have been identified in South Africa but do not appear to be regular parasites of racing pigeons.

Pathogenicity

The blood-sucking worms burrow into the intestinal mucosa causing catarrhal to haemorrhagic enteritis with ulceration and necrosis. This predisposes the bird to secondary infections and heavy losses may occur.

Symptoms

Depending on the degree of infestation the symptoms may vary from a puffed-up bird with mild lassitude to a very sick pigeon with anorexia, severe diarrhoea, excessive thirst, vomiting, rapid loss of weight, blood in the faeces and death. Loss of control over movement is sometimes seen.

Pathology

Post mortem examination reveals dehydration, anaemia, haemor-rhagic enteritis and necrotic ulcers in the bowel. Large sections of bowel mucosa may be sloughed off.

Diagnosis

The presence of thin-shelled eggs, usually in the morula stage, is diagnostic.

Control and Treatment

Because of the short lifecycle, sanitation is absolutely essential. Lofts are cleaned regularly (daily) and wire bottom cages are used with success. Food and water containers must be kept covered and never soiled by droppings. Treatment with piperazine, levamisole and thiabendazole is effective.

2.3. CAPILLARIA SPP. (Hairworm)

The hairworm is probably the most important internal parasite occuring in pigeons, as its presence is not readily diagnosed by the average fancier, leading him to treat for other forms of enteritis. Rare in South Africa before the 1960s, they have subsequently been found in all the provinces, presumably having been intro-duced from Europe. In Germany it is estimated that 50% of the pigeons are infested.

Comparing the relative sizes of Coccidia oocysts (large), eggs of Tetramares Americana, Capillaria species, Ascaridia Columbae and Acuaria Spiralis (enlarged 100 times).

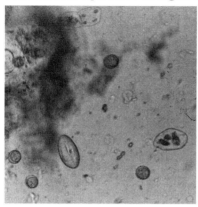

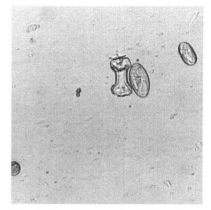

Coccidia and Tetrameres eggs.

Coccidia, Tetrameres and Acuria eggs (digestive material resembles an apple core).

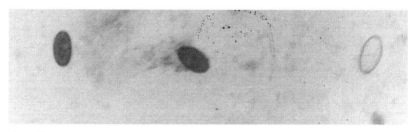

Capillaria and Tetrameres eggs.

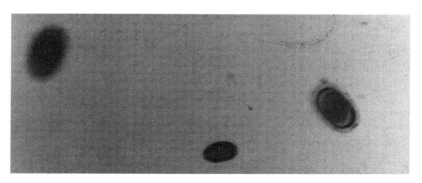

Capillaria and Ascaridia eggs.

Epidemiology

Three species are recognised in pigeons, viz. Capillaria obsignata, C.contorta and C. caudinflata, the latter being the only one that does not have a direct lifecycle, having the earthworm as interme- diate host. As racing pigeons do not generally consume earth- worms, hairworms in pigeons are considered to have a direct lifecycle, completed, under favourable conditions, in about two weeks. This can cause an infestation to spread very rapidly to all the occupants of a loft.

The eggs are excreted in the droppings and under favourable conditions of heat and moisture, larvae develop inside the egg within one week. When the pigeon consumes the embryonated egg (on contaminated grain or water) the larvae excysts, develops to maturity and lays eggs. Eggs remain viable outside the host for seven months under cool moist conditions.

C. obsignata is not host-specific and infected chickens can be a source of infection for pigeons.

Pathogenesis

Hairworms produce moderate to severe enteritis. The excysted larvae penetrate the intestinal lining, causing extensive primary damage. Secondary damage is caused by invading bacteria. Adult worms produce a toxin which causes debilitation and listlessness.

Symptoms

Diarrhoea is noticed with faeces caked on the vent feathers. The droppings are loose, dark green and very tacky. The birds do not eat, rapidly lose weight, sit hunched up and are unwilling to move. Anaemia is seen in the membranes of the throat and tongue and in the eye colour. Often the first signs are missed and when first spotted, the bird may already be extremely ill. Deaths can occur in both adult and young birds.

Pathology and Diagnosis

Post-mortem examination reveals a reddened and thickened intes- tine with sloughing of epithelium and epithelial plugs in the lumen in severe cases. These are easily mistaken for a bacterial or viral enteritis as the worms are not readily visible without the use of a microscope. Microscopical examination of the faeces, reveals

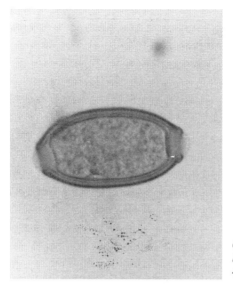

*Capillaria egg, note
bipolar cap (enlarged
400 times).*

numerous bipolar-capped eggs. The worms are seen if a light
scraping is made of the intestinal lining and the harvested material placed between two glass slides, spread thinly and examined
against a plain background. The worms appear as coiled threads,
from 10 to 26 mm in length.

In the live bird the diagnosis is made by the identification of the
typical eggs in the faeces.

Treatment and Control

Methyridine was the first drug used successfully against hairworms. Levamisole (Tramisol) given per os is effective against
both hairworms and roundworms. Febantel, fenbendazole and
cambendazole have also been used with success but great care
must be exercised owing to their toxicity for pigeons. Ivermectin
injectible has given excellent results.

Control consists of absolute sanitation. Regular (daily) cleaning
is essential and sand or ground floors cannot be tolerated. Blanket
treatment of all new introductions to the loft is recommended.
Screening of faeces is done by a veterinary surgeon or pathology
laboratory on a fresh sample.

2.4. CESTODES (Tapeworms)

The tapeworm species found in pigeons are; Hymenolepis,

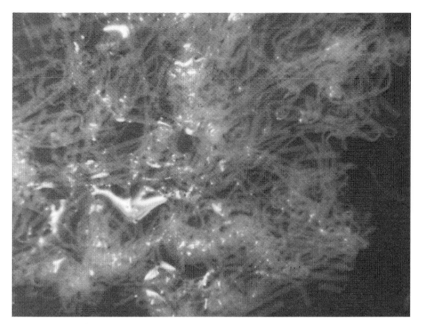

Tapeworms, Raillietina Bonini. This is one teaspoonful removed and washed, several teaspoonfuls can infest a single pigeon.

Davainea, Aporina, Railiettina or Contugia. They occur in pigeons throughout the world and are not usually considered to be of much importance. Many anecdotes are told about pigeons in a race, arriving at the loft in winning time, with a tapeworm hanging from the cloaca. These incidents occur on shorter and faster races, when not so much effort is required from the birds; In long and hard races infested pigeons will find it difficult to perform well. The sporadic finding of tapeworms in pigeons has not been a regular feature of diagnosis.

Lifecycle

All cestodes have an intermediate lifecycle, with a variety of inter-mediate hosts, such as arthropods, molluscs (snails) and annelids. Cestodes have a scolex (head) and body. The scolex attaches to the intestinal lining, feeds and grows to maturity. When sexual matu-rity is reached and fertilization has occurred the proglottids (ripe segments – filled with eggs) are detached continuously and excreted in the faeces to release the eggs. The eggs are taken up by the intermediate host (snail), and develops an embryo, which

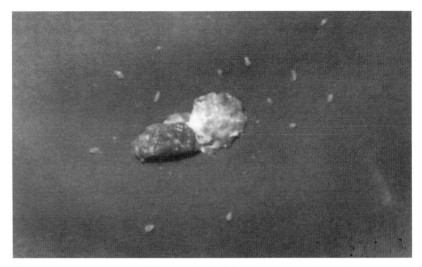

Tapeworm segments (Raillietina Bonini) leaving a dropping within minutes of being exreted.

penetrates the intestinal wall of the snail, developing to a cysticercus (bladderworm or measle). At this stage the snail is infective and if swallowed by a pigeon, the scolex inside the cysticercus evaginates, attaches to the intestinal wall of the pigeon and repeats the cycle, which takes about six weeks.

Pathogenicity

Damage occurs in three ways. The attaching scolex causes loss of intestinal villi, predisposing to secondary infection. Through consumption of available feedstuffs by the worm, the host is denied nutrition. In addition the waste products of the worms are irritant and interfere with normal digestion.

Symptoms

Racing performance is decreased, the pigeons lack condition and do not thrive, seeming to lose vigour when subjected to stress. Mortalities are not usually seen.

   Gravid proglottids may be seen leaving the droppings, which may be firm and normal in colour. A few minutes after being voided the segments crawl to the surface of the dropping, from where they attempt to leave it. They are small (approximately 3 x 1mm), a pale fleshy colour and as many as 20 or 30 proglottids may be recovered from one dropping.

In other species, once the proglottid is expelled with the faeces, it secretes its eggs in the dropping.

Pathology and Diagnosis

In the live pigeon diagnosis is based upon demonstration of segments or eggs in the faeces.

On autopsy, loss of condition and mild enteritis may be the only pathological changes. The worms are seen in the intestine, but some cestodes are so thin that they are not readily apparent and easy to miss. If the intestinal content is picked up with a fine tweezer, it will appear tenacious and thready. Upon washing and viewing against a dark background, the worms become apparent.

Treatment and control

Many drugs have been used successfully for the control of tape-worms in human and animal medicine. Unfortunately very little work has been done on cestodes in pigeons and birds and we have to experiment with medications used in other fields. We have found Niclosamide (Lintex) and Praziquantel (Droncit) to be effective.

The lifecycle of the tapeworms must be broken and, as pigeons avidly seek out snails they must be denied all access to the living areas of the molluscs. Failure to achieve this, results in immediate reinfestation.

The pigeons must, at no time, be allowed access to grassed areas or other areas where snails are found. The most satisfactory control consists in keeping pigeons in the loft when not flying.

2.5. TREMATODES (flukes)

Although not commonly encountered, many species of flukes have been identified in pigeons. Amongst others are Echinostoma, Echinoparyphium, Hypoderaeum, Brachylaemus, Apatemom and Cotylurus. Flukes are flat leaflike organisms, varying in size with many species exceeding one centimetre in length. They parasitise any part of the body but in pigeons the majority are found in the small intestine and caecum.

Lifecycle

The known lifecycles of flukes are rather involved, part being spent as a free living miracidium and later again as free living cercaricum, both in standing or slow-flowing water and one, two or more intermediate hosts are involved. For this reason flukes are not likely to become a serious problem in a well-managed pigeon loft. We have not personally seen pigeons affected with flukes, but have had cases described that closely resemble and could well have been fluke infestations.

Pathogenicity

Severe enteritis has been described with up to 600 flukes found on autopsy. Mortalities have been caused by Echinostoma revolutum and Echinoparyphium paraulum.

Symptoms and Diagnosis

The symptoms are those of an enteritis including lassitude, inappetence, thirst, diarrhoea and progressive weakness. Diagnosis is made on finding the eggs of the flukes in the faeces of the pigeon.

Treatment and Control

Carbon tetrachloride and tetrachlorethylene have been recommended but many of the newer helminticides are probably more effective. Control is essential and the lifecycle must be interrupted by keeping the birds inside the loft, or laying dry the wet areas in which the parasite passes through its miracidial and cercarial stages. Ponds and dams can be cleared of snails by adding copper sulphate to the water in concentrations not less than one in 500,000. This will be detrimental to other water life, including fish.

B. ECTOPARASITES

The external parasites of pigeons are generally well-known and most are easy to control. As they are readily apparent, an undue amount of emphasis is often placed upon their presence, with the result that the birds are sometimes subjected to excessive antiparasitic eradication programmes.

On the other hand, the presence of ectoparasites on pigeons is an indication of the standard of management and though not necessarily detrimental to the birds, it reflects negatively on the care bestowed, and questions whether other, essential functions are performed with the necessary diligence and discipline.

1. Lice

Many species of lice can infest pigeons but as they do not occur in great numbers under good hygienic conditions, they are not considered to be of great significance.

The lifecycle of most pigeon lice is the same, being completed on the bird. The eggs, known as nits, are laid and attached to the feather shaft. When hatched, they produce nymphs, which feed on feathers, skin scales, tissue fluid or blood and go through various stages to become adult lice. After mating these produce eggs and the whole lifecycle is completed in four to five weeks.

At present the full significance of lice on pigeons has yet to be fully understood. We do not know for certain what role they play in the transmission of disease, nor can it be determined how much irritation they cause. In chickens egg-laying is reduced, and we assume that racing performance in pigeons, is affected.

1.1 Columbicola columbae (Slender louse)

Columbicola columbae is readily identified, as the long slender feather louse, easily seen on the primary wing feathers when held against the light. Feather lice are reported to cause damage to the feathers and it is claimed by some that the pin-holes sometimes seen in the flags of the primary feathers are due to feather lice. We have found no evidence to support these claims and believe that feather lice do not physically damage the feathers. The parasite is very common but even when occurring in great numbers, it is not detrimental to the bird's health.

1.2 Campanulotes (Gonicotes) bidentatus, the Small Louse is mainly found on the rump, particularly when the rump feathers are brushed in reverse direction. They are seen singly or in pairs (large female, small male).

As they live on feather dust, the amount of damage caused, is questionable. They are only able to survive for about six days off the host.

Other lice are regularly but rarely found on pigeons when the management is below standard. Some biting lice (Mallophaga) of poultry are bloodsuckers and can cause a drastic drop in egg production, anaemia and death. Should pigeons be the host, severe effects could be reflected in their lack of performance.

The spread of lice amongst pigeons occurs from close contact, such as in training and racing panniers. Increased parasitism is also noted during the warmer summer months.

2. Mites (acarids)

Mites are smaller than lice and are generally only seen under magnification. A good magnifying glass will greatly facilitate the examination. Much controversy and misunderstanding exists about mites.

Many fanciers claim to have seen red mites on their pigeons but this is unlikely and is probably a mistaken identification for feather mites. The red mite only visits the pigeon to feed at night, hiding in dark corners the rest of its life. All mites, except the red mite and harvest mite, complete their lifecycle on the host.

2.1. Red mite (Dermanyssus gallinae)

Being an avid bloodsucker the red mite is capable of causing severe and fatal anaemia. They attack their host at night only and hide in cracks, crevices and nests during the day. They are controlled by the regular and thorough use of an insecticidal wash or spray on the floors, walls, roof and in the nestboxes. Though the life-cycle of the red mite can be completed in only seven days, the parasite can live without a meal for up to five months, so a disused loft must be cleaned and disinfected before repopulation takes place.

The history is typically those of sick pigeons with listlessness, reduced willingness to train, lack of performance, increased losses and general malaise. Anaemia is the only symptom but may be so severe as to cause death. When the birds are heard to be restless, stamping their feet at night, red mite must be suspected. If a light is suddenly brought on, the engorged mites can be seen as small red specks, scurrying away from the birds to their hiding places.

Red mites have been shown to transmit various virus diseases. They also attack human beings, causing skin lesions.

2.2. Feather mites (Megnignia columbae and Falculifer spp.)

Six species of feather mites have been found on pigeons. They are found on virtually all untreated birds in great numbers. The full lifecycle is completed on the pigeon, where they live on feather dust and skin scales. Although not generally regarded as harmful, the nymphs of some species (e.g. Falculifer corrutus) will enter the subcutaneous or peritracheal tissues, causing physical discomfort.

Feather mites are smaller than red mites, and can only be seen properly when magnified. The feather shaft mite (Falculifer rostratus) is slightly larger and is found on the shaft and web of flight feathers, adjacent to the shaft. It seems to prefer white feathers and can be seen particularly on the underside of the wing, when examined against the light.

Transmission between lofts occurs through the close contact of the birds in racing and training panniers.

Treatment consists of dipping or spraying the birds with a malathion solution (e.g.Duramitex) or dusting with a carbamate-containing powder (e.g. Karbadust). Pigeons have won races and performed well within days of being treated with the above insecticides, indicating the safety of the products.

2.3. Scaly leg mite (Cnemidocoptes mutans)

Scaly leg mites are flat mites with stubby legs living exclusively in the subcutaneous tissues of the legs and feet, where they live on blood serum and cutaneous tissues. They burrow in and under the skin, causing irritation, swelling and inflammation. The skin becomes hard, crusty and swollen with calcareous scabs, causing difficulty in walking.

Treatment consists of soaking the feet and legs in a bland oil, which softens the scabs, making their removal easier after which a suitable insecticide e.g. Malathion is applied. A few treatments will usually be sufficient. Although frequently seen in chickens, the complaint is rare in pigeons.

2.4. Quill mite (Syringophilus columbae)

Very seldom seen. Quill mites are found inside the quills of the larger wing and tail flights, causing them to break, leaving only the stumps. The mites are rarely seen. Treatment consists of a suitable dip using malathion or carbaryl.

2.5. Airsac mite (Cytodites nudus)

Airsac mites live in the airsacs and airways, especially the trachea, but may penetrate to the liver and kidneys. They are tiny mites appearing as small white granules in the airsacs and are easily missed on examination. They cause respiratory problems with anorexia, loss of weight and weakness. The birds sneeze and make whistling respiratory sounds. In severe cases the airsacs contain a tacky liquid and pneumonia and aerocystitis result. The diagnosis is made by finding the mite eggs in the faeces, or by demonstrating the mites in the airsacs at autopsy.

Treatment is difficult, but a vaporising dichlorvos bar (Vapona), hung in the loft and giving off miticidal fumes, may be sufficient.

Fairly common in poultry and canaries, the airsac mite is not readily found in racing pigeon lofts.

2.6. Nasal mite (Neonyssus columbae, Neonyssus melloi, Speleognathus striatus)

These mites cause irritation of the nasal cavity with a resultant wet nose (dd ornithosis). Treatment is suggested as for airsac mite.

2.7. Depluming itch mite (Neocnemidocoptes laevis)

Very rare in racing pigeons. Found at the base and on the shaft of the feathers inside the follicle particularly on the neck. The mites can be seen in the thickened shafts of the feathers, causing premature shedding and breakages at skin level. The mites cause severe stress to the bird.

Treatment is by injection of ivermectin.

2.8. Harvest mite (Trombicula autumnalis)

Only the larvae of the harvest mite cause problems. Although not a common parasite of pigeons, they are included because straw, which is occasonally used as bedding in pigeon lofts, can be infected with harvest mites. Serious consequences result if mites are introduced. The mites have a nasty bite, causing pruritus and secondary infection, severe enough to kill chickens. The mites also attack other animals and humans, causing intense itchiness and leaving large raised welts.

2.9. Other mites

The other mites sometimes found on pigeons are not common, and too little is known of their life-cycle, pathology or treatment to warrant inclusion.

3. Pigeon Fly (Pseudolynchia canariensis)

The pigeon fly (louse fly) is a hard, flat, dark-grey parasite, 6mm long, resembling a sheep ked. It is found in most countries with a moderate climate. Considered a nuisance by fanciers, it can be difficult to control. When pigeons are handled, the flies are felt as they scuttle about under the feathers. When flying, they move at great speed from one bird to another, or to a spot nearby.

Lifecycle

The fly feeds on pigeons, causing painful bites and sucking blood. (They also bite man). Pale creamy/white eggs (3 mm x 2.5 mm) are laid in dark corners or in the nests, developing into black pupae after a few hours. The black, match-head size pupae can be seen in unused nest boxes or on the floor when nesting material is removed. The pupae mature in about one month to release the adult flies which live about 40 to 45 days, the females laying four to five eggs during this time. Deep litter in a loft creates a favourable breeding environment for pigeon flies.

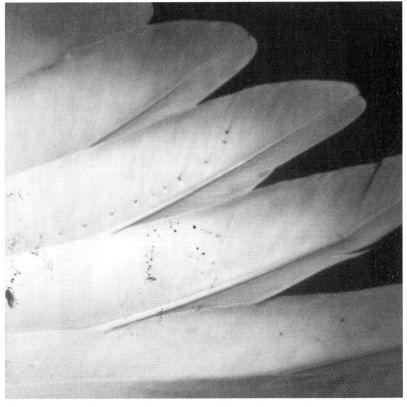

Pinpricks on the primary flights caused by thge pigeon fly puncturing the young, rolled-up feather sheath in search of blood.

Pathogenesis

The bites of the fly are irritant to the pigeon, causing disturbed rest and resultant difficulty in achieving top racing form. P. canariensis transmits the blood protozoon, Haemoproteus columbae, which causes pseudomalaria in pigeons. The parasite is also responsible for the mechanical transmission of disease, particularly pigeon pox.

Control

Control is easy if basic routines are followed;

- Regular cleaning of the loft, including shelves, corners, perches and nest boxes. Unused nest boxes may be quite clean – except for a few fly eggs, maturing in a corner.

- Pigeon fly introductions are prevented with a six-monthly wetting of the inside of the loft, using a long-acting contact insecticide. Wetting must be thorough and cover every square centimetre in the loft, after which the loft is allowed to dry thoroughly before the pigeons are returned. Wetting the loft via washing is more effective. Sprayed solutions are prevented from wetting the loft by a fine water-repellent layer of feather dust, removed by physical washing.

It is not necessary to use insecticides on the birds and this should be avoided to prevent toxic reactions. Dust and manure swept from the loft must be destroyed or removed from the vicinity, preventing newly-hatched flies from rehabitating the loft.

We have successfully used permethrins (Coopex, Ambush) and chlorpyrifos (Dursban).

4. Bugs (Bedbug – Cimex lectularius)

Various bugs have been described on pigeons around the world but only the common bedbug is regularly seen. It is found where the loft management is below standard.

Eggs are laid in cracks and crevices. Nymphs hatch and moult five times before developing into adults to complete the life cycle, a process which is completed in six to ten weeks under favourable circumstances. Nymphs hide in dark secluded areas (under nest-pans) during the day, coming out at night to feed, needing a meal of blood to progress to the next stage. Adult bedbugs can exist in empty lofts or buildings for 12 months without feeding.

Control

Bug control involves thorough cleaning, followed by spraying the premises and equipment where the bugs hide. Recommended insecticides include malathion (Duramitex, Malasol), permethrins (Coopex, Ambush) and chlorpyrifos (Dursban).

5. Ticks

We have not seen ticks on pigeons but, according to the literature, they are regularly encountered in Europe, America and other areas of the world.

Argas persicus is reported from Belgium, USA, S. America and Australia to occur on pigeons. Other species of Argas, Ixodes, Ornithodoros, Dermacentor, Amblyomma, Hyalomma and Rhipicephalus are reported from the rest of the world.

Control

Control measures are similar to the ones for removing bugs. Individual ticks can be removed by directly applying nail polish or tobacco oil to the parasite. All grass and vegetation surrounding the loft where the birds may make contact, is removed or severely trimmed.

6. Mosquitoes

Most pigeon fanciers are aware of mosquitoes in their lofts at certain times. If few in numbers, little damage is done, but large numbers can cause loss of condition and form, in addition to transmitting disease.

Lifecycle

Eggs are laid in water or on floating vegetable matter – each of the many species having its own requirements. Some species may lay their eggs only in fresh rain water, others in stagnant water or at the edges of streams and some species even require salt water. The hatching larvae take 7 to 16 days to mature, depending mainly on the temperature of the water in which they live.

Pathogenesis

Large numbers of mosquitoes in a loft can cause enough disturbance to the pigeons to prevent successful racing. Anaemia can
occur under such conditions.

Mosquitoes are more dangerous because they transmit diseases
– both biologically and mechanically, to man and all animals.

Mosquitoes are the vectors of pigeon pox and the disease regularly occurs in those lofts where vaccination is not carried out.
Some diseases of pigeons are thought to be spread by mosquitoes,
but this has yet to be confirmed.

Control

In order to destroy the breeding places, it is essential that all
watery areas near the loft are laid dry or covered with a thin layer
of oil.

Where practical, mosquito netting is fitted to the loft openings.
Contact insecticides are available for use on walls and ceilings to
control house flies and these appear to be useful for controlling
mosquitoes, though control has been complicated by resistance
developing in mosquitoes. Fumigating dichlorvos bars (Vapona),
hung in the loft, have been used with some success where the loft
is not too open.

Chapter 8

Neoplasms

As in other animals, including man, abnormal growth of tissue occasionally occurs, resulting in the formation of neoplasms, which can be malignant or benign. They usually occur on an individual basis in older specimens and, because the average age of a race team seldom exceeds three, they are not of great significance in the race team. Breeding pigeons, however tend to be older before their worth is discovered and the loss of individual specimens can make a large difference to a team of stock birds. All systems are affected although skin tumours, being more readily observed, tend to receive more attention.

As in other species the etiology of tumours in pigeons is largely unknown. Viruses have been identified as causing some forms of

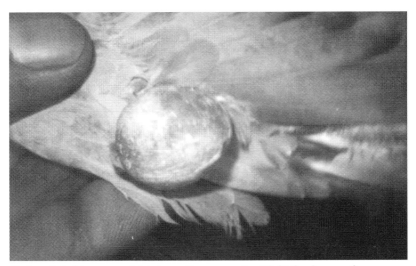

Peduculated tumour which is easily removed with little chance of recurrence.

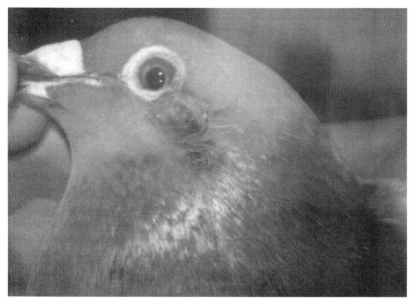

Superficial benign tumour of the face. Easily removable at this stage but if treatment is delayed lack of healthy skin will prevent the wound closing.

cancer in chickens and probaby do the same in pigeons. No studies have shown this but we can assume that similar tumours have similar etiologies.

Benign (non-malignant) growths

It seems that these are seen more often on the outside of the body. Growths that occur internally tend to be more malignant. External growths are generally easy to remove, making their early identification and treatment a viable proposition.

The single biggest mistake that fanciers make, is to wait too long. Numerous instances can be quoted where a salvageable condition caused the death of the bird because the fancier delayed treatment. This is particularly true of external, benign growths but applies equally to some malignant growths. Lack of healthy tissue to fill the space previously occupied by the neoplasm, is another result of delaying surgery.

Blood warts or Atypial pox

Blood warts occur fairly regularly, though never as an outbreak, even though the pox virus is apparently causative. One or two birds, usually young birds or yearlings, not having built an immunity, are affected. Wart-like lesions appear on the pigeon, usually singly but occasionally a few in number. The lesions are black, vary in size from a pea to a walnut and bleed very easily. After three to four weeks they regress spontaneously, after which no more lesions are seen. Typical pox particles are seen by means of electronmicroscopy and confirms the etiology of an atypial pox virus.

The conditon occurs irrespective of a simultaneous pox outbreak or previous pox vaccination. It has not yet been established whether it is caused by an aberrant pox virus (mutant possibly) or an abnormal tissue reaction. Surgical removal is not necessary, as spontaneous healing takes place but injured blood warts bleed profusely, and pigeons have bled to death from haemorrhaging blood warts. Isolation in a protected environment is preferable. Following natural drying of the lesion, the blood wart drops off and complete recovery occurs.

Lipoma

Lipoma is an abnormal localised accumulation of fat cells, always benign. It is normally situated outside the body and has to be differentiated from abnormal generalised fatty accumulation, which appears to be genetic. Genetic fatty accumulation occurs both internally and externally and regrows upon section. Only the larger fatty masses can be removed and the internal fat is too intimately interwoven with normal tissue, particularly the intestine, to permit sectioning.

Xanthoma

Xanthomas occur in mammals, including man, where they form yellowish plaques in the skin. In pigeons, xanthomas are recognisable as thickened areas of skin, strongly coloured yellow. They occur mainly in the ventral abdominal area where they can be readily excisd. Xanthomas, if left unattended, are unsightly and interfere with breeding. Once unmanageable proportions are reached, not enough healthy skin may remain to cover the large defect.

Malignant neoplasms

Malignant neoplasms in pigeons are mainly found internally and are usually diagnosed when operative procedures are attempted.

External malignant growths are frequently invasive of surrounding tissues and cannot be operated without causing serious disfigurement. Not many malignancies are brought for examination or treatment probably because of the rapid nature of cancer in pigeons. Often a fancier will wait as long as possible and will seek help only when breeding is no longer possible. Another cause for the paucity of cases brought in is that most of the birds are at an advanced age and can be replaced. It is some times not considered worth the trouble and expense to subject the bird to examination and surgical treatment, when, it is estimated, little can usually be accomplished anyway. Such bird is rather suppressed.

When the cancer invades a wing, amputation of the limb is a viable option in a valuable bird. Though left unable to fly, the bird can continue breeding in a low nestbox if food and water are placed within reach. If the life of the pigeon is only temporarily prolonged, any offspring gained in the post-operative period, makes the effort worthwhile. Postponement of the procedure, however, often leads to an inoperable state.

The more common internal malignant neoplasms in pigeons are usually very rapidly growing, difficult to diagnose, impossible to treat and fatal. They are invariably of the lymphosarcoma, lymphoid leukosis or adenocarcinoma type. Internal tumours of the abdomen can usually be palpated and, if large, cause respiratory symptoms. They can be confused with egg binding, retained yolk, large internal haemorrhage, abdominal abscess, abdominal aspergillosis etc, but X-ray and laparoscopy will reveal the true condition.

Most of the malignancies that occur in mammals are probably found in pigeons, and all organs are likely affected. However, the laxness of fanciers to provide cases, lack of proper identification and administration by central laboratories, coincide to make the knowledge about malignant tumours scarce and incomplete. Much more research is needed in this field and it awaits the enthusiasm of a qualified scientist.

Chapter 9

Toxins
and poisons

A poison is a substance that, when absorbed or in contact with live tissue, injures or destroys life and health. A toxin is a poisonous substance of animal or plant origin and the term is used particularly for a poison produced by micro organisms.

Our store of knowledge regarding the pigeon's susceptibility to various poisons is limited. Though allegations are often levied by fanciers, particularly against a variety of plants, little scientific evidence of poisoning is recorded. Some of these claims are noted, so that one day a complete and corroborated record may exist.

A well-managed team of pigeons is unlikely to be poisoned. However lack of knowledge or carelessness can lead to severe losses. An aware fancier is always on the lookout for the possibility of poisoning, particularly when their birds are bathing or foraging, even if only in the garden in front of the loft. When dramatic cases of poisoning occur and numerous pigeons die, non-affected fanciers are quick to correct problems in their own situations. But when the poisoned birds are only slightly out of sorts, poisoning is often not suspected and heavy losses may occur during races. I believe that this occurs more frequently than suspected or reported.

The prevention of poisoning must always be a top priority; treatment is a salvage effort and takes second place. Consequently little is known about antidotes, treatment and post-poisoning care, which are direct derivatives of mammalian methods. Concentration must centre on recognition of dangerous practices and removal of suspicious substances and situations.

1. Plant poisoning

Many toxic plants growing in today's gardens would, if fed to pigeons, be poisonous. However, toxicity of a substance to pigeons is related to the likelihood of that substance being eaten by pigeons. If pigeons are not liable to eat a specific plant or its seed voluntarily, it cannot justifiably be reckoned to be toxic for them. For example, Nerium Oleander, the Rose of Ceylon, of which all the parts i.e. leaves, flowers, seeds and stems are highly poisonous cannot be classified as toxic to pigeons as there is no part that the birds are likely to consume. Toxicity of plants varies tremendously, depending on the stage of growth and their physical position within environment.

1.1. SESBANIA PUNICEA.

Originally exported from South America as an ornamental plant, Sesbania is a deciduous shrub of the legume family, producing red or orange flowers in early summer. Seeds are formed in pods, which burst open when ripe. The seeds, flowers and leaves of the plant are lethal to such animals as sheep, rabbits, guinea pigs, chickens, turkeys, ducks, pigeons and other birds. Pigeons eat the seeds voraciously and seven seeds may be sufficient to cause mortality. Toxicity of the seeds varies widely.

Symptoms and Pathology

Symptoms of poisoning include vomiting, depression, diarrhoea and death. Pigeons appear to have respiratory problems.

On autopsy haemorrhages are seen in the proventriculus. The presence of seeds in the crop and/or gizzard makes the diagnosis irrefutable.

Treatment and Control

No effective treatment is known. Control rests with the removal of all Sesbania bushes from the vicinity of the loft.

1.2. HYDRANGEA MACROPHYLLA

Hydrangea macrophylla, the Christmas flower, is a popular flowering bush, which has for many years been believed to be toxic to pigeons. The pigeons apparently feed on the green buds before new leaves appear, vomit and die.

We have done some small trials, feeding fresh buds to adult birds. but have not been able to reproduce signs of poisoning with buds. However, one whole medium-sized leaf fed to a pigeon killed it within 36 hours. It would be safer prevent to pigeons having access to leaves, developing and fully grown.

1.3. RAPE (BRASSICA NAPUS)

The seeds of various Brassicae spp, particularly rape, sometimes used in pigeon feed, contain a goitrogenic factor and mustard oils (alkyl isothiocyanates), and are harmful. Though not usually fed in large enough quantities to cause explicit poisoning, other seeds exist with equally beneficial properties (rich in fat) and it is recommended that rape seed be excluded "in toto" from pigeon rations.

2. Insecticides

Deaths have occurred when untested insecticides are used on pigeons, they represent a terrible waste, as most of such tragedies can so easily have been avoided.

Whenever a new untried insecticide is to be used for dipping, bathing or powdering the birds, the fancier ought always to do a trial run. A few, less valuable, birds are treated in the desired manner and observed for 24 hours. If no undesirable side-effects follow, the rest may be done. Although troublesome, this procedure prevents the heartache and self-reproach that follows when a loft is destroyed by a singular irresponsible action. It happens regularly.

There are three main ways in which pigeons are affected by insecticides.

- The insecticide, aimed against lice, mites or pigeon flies, is applied to the birds in the form of a dip or spray usually in incorrect dilution.

- Pigeons are fed grains that have either become accidentally contaminated with poison or have been treated with insecticides.

- Foraging pigeons consume poisoned grains, or poisoned water. Dead, poisoned insects, if eaten in large quantities, can cause poisoning.

The insecticides for use on pigeons or by which pigeons are poisoned, consist mainly of chlorinated hydrocarbons, organophosphates or pyrethrins.

CHLORINATED HYDROCARBON INSECTICIDES

Examples include DDT, DDD, Dylan, Methoxychlor, Perthane, BHC (incl Lindane), Aldrin, Dieldrin, Endrin, Isodrin, Chlordane, Strobane and Toxaphene. DDT, BHC, Dieldrin and Chlordane are the most common.

Because of their danger in the environment, the chlorinated hydrocarbons were withdrawn from the market several years ago. Some members of the group, though, are still available and pigeons are occasionally poisoned by them. None are recommended for use on pigeons.

Symptoms

They are diffuse stimulants of the central nervous system, therefore the chlorinated hydrocarbons cause predominantly neuromuscular signs. However pigeons may die without showing any overt signs of nervous disorder. The more usual symptoms include diarrhoea, vomiting, anorexia, trembling, waddling gait, convulsions, wing-standing (supporting its own weight on the wings and not using the legs), paralysis and death.

Autopsy

Generalised severe congestion of the carcase and all the organs, is the only change regularly seen. Haemorrhages sometimes occur in the heart and other organs. The intestines may show signs of enteritis. There usually are no other specific changes.

Treatment

In cases where chlorinated hydrocarbon poison has been taken orally, it is important not to administer an oily purgative, as these insecticides are fat-soluble and the treatment enhances absorption. The use of a saline purgative is recommended.

When poisoning has occurred through skin contact, attempts are made to remove the insecticide, by washing in soapy luke-warm water. No specific antidote is available against the chlorinated hydrocarbons.

ORGANOPHOSPHATE INSECTICIDES.

Examples include Chlorthion, DDVP, Demeton, Diazinon, Dimefox, Dimethoate, Dimethylparathion, Neguvon (Dipterex)

(Dylox), Dursban (Chlorpyrifos), EPN, Etrolene (Dow 57), HETP, Malathion, Metasystox, Mipafox, Parathion, Potasan (Asuntol), Ruelene, Schradan, Sulfotepp, TEPP

Insecticides in common usage are: Diazinon, Neguvon, Dursban, Malathion (least toxic, used on birds as Duramitex), Parathion, Metasystox and Asuntol.

Organophosphorous insecticides exert their action by inhibition of cholinesterase.

Symptoms

Affected pigeons show trembling, vomiting, tripping over feet, hypersensitivity, diarrhoea, weakness, open-mouth breathing, resting on sternum, waddling gait, incoordination, curling of toes, sitting on hocks, droopy eyelids, closed eyes, depression, lying on chest, coma and death.

Severely poisoned birds may be seen lying on the floor unable to walk or fly and may die without showing any of the other signs. Others may lie with wings outstretched and head trown back, eyes open or closed.

Depression and respiratory embarassment (raised back, pumping keel) is often seen. Usually only one or two of the symptoms are seen per pigeon and not all birds, affected with the same poison, show the same changes.

Autopsy

Dead birds are usually found on their sternums, with outstretched wings and uncurled toes.

The autopsy varies; it is essentially negative, or with major changes, particularly haemorrhagic, and all stages in between..

A dehydrated carcase is often seen with subcutaneous haemorrhages and a crop that can be full or empty, depending on whether the bird vomited. The liver is dark, enlarged and congested. Haemorrhages in the spleen, enlarged to two to three times the normal and the kidney, swollen and dark red, are common. The pancreas is dark-pink. Haemorrhages are seen in the lungs and trachea.

Treatment

A few products are registered for use against the organophosphates. Valuable birds can be saved with intensive treatment. Pigeons that have recuperated from poisoning, recover their full racing and breeding potentials.

Atropine sulphate is recommended in the literature, but we have seen little improvement following its use. It is given every 30 minutes till improvement is noted and then every two hours. (0.25ml of 0.5% soln)

2-PAM or Toxogonin may be used with good success. The injection (2 ml of a 2.5 % solution) is repeated every four to six hours. Response in seen in 5-10 minutes. Repeated doses are required, allowing the body time to detoxify and eliminate the poison.

In all cases the birds are in a state of shock and supportive treatment, in the form of sucutaneous fluid administration and heated cages, are an essential part of successful treatment. In severe cases steroid therapy is given as an adjunct to the above.

Pigeons that have been dipped and have shown symptoms, take five to seven days to recover to the point where no more symptoms are seen. Full recovery to a useful state requires a long recuperative period.

PERMETHRINS

Permethrins, the active principles in pyrethrum, are made from vegetable material and are the least toxic of all the insecticides. Effective use is made of them in controlling pigeon fly (Pseudolynchia canariensis). Best known products include Coopex and Ambush (agricultural).

CARBAMATES

Carbamates inhibit cholinesterase action. Best known products are; methomyl (Lannate – Du Pont); propoxur (Baygon – Bayer AG) and carbaryl (Sevin – Union Carbide, Karbadust – Exceder, Karbadip Spray – Rumevite).

They are normally available as powder preparations, in which form they are not liable to cause poisoning in pigeons.

2.1. Dips and sprays.

This form of poisoning is the most common. It occurs suddenly and is the more devastating because it happens through a fancier's own folly, and he is overcome by remorse and grief. A whole loft can be eradicated.

Following the correct procedure, a trial is first done on less valuable birds whenever a new dip, bath, spray or powder is used. By waiting 24 hours for possible side-effects to manifest themselves, a whole team of birds might be saved. It is a troublesome method, but preferable to killing favourite pigeons and up-and-coming champions! The safe alternative is to stay with tried and tested products and to leave experimentation to someone else.

Though it is not widely recognised, it is important to know that insecticides are absorbed through the skin (percutaneous absorbtion). For one's own protection, waterproof gloves are worn whenever the birds are dipped. Though they do not drink of the poison, pigeons can be fatally poisoned when dipped. Skin contact is sufficient for a lethal quantity of poison to be absorbed. We have seen colonies exterminated within 48 hours from skin-absorbed insecticide poisoning.

Dips are more likely than powder to cause poisoning, as contact between the dilution and the skin is closer and absorption is better. Most poisoning invariably occurs following incorrect use of dips, when either the wrong insecticide is used or the concentration is incorrect.

Pigeons are not liable to bathe in poisoned bathwater because of their highly-developed sense of smell. Very little percutaneous absorption takes place from powders.

2.2. Poisoned grains

It does not happen regularly that pigeons are fed poisoned feed, but it can be a devastating and difficult problem to solve. The fancier has no control over the grains prior to their arrival at his loft and he must trust the commonsense of the merchants who deal in stock feeds and the farmers who produce them.

Case history: Some years ago I received a report from an area where the pigeons of local fanciers were dying suddenly and mysteriously. The birds were locked in the loft, fine and healthy. They'd be fed and one or two hours later two or three pigeons would die acutely. The others in the same loft would be well and healthy and carry on with their normal activities. For the next day or two, there would be no losses, until one or two more would suddenly die after being fed. This was happening to various fanciers in the town, many eventually losing up to 60% of their stock; as did keepers of other birds and poultry.

When diazinon poisoning was finally diagnosed from a feed sample, the source of poison was traced to the local grain merchant. He had spilled poison in the storage room, cleared up the spillage but the poison that had penetrated the feed sacks, had contaminated the grains in contact with the sack. Once tipped out of the sack, they were mixed with clean grains resulting in the sporadic and mysterious losses.

2.3. Foraging and gardening

For many years it has been a standard practice to protect seed grains against insect attack by using insecticide. Should these be discovered by foraging pigeons, trouble can result.

Pigeons are not by nature solely grain eaters and avidly devour small snails, wood lice (pill bugs or sow bugs) and other insects. If these are poisoned and eaten, they can in turn, cause poisoning.

It is to be born in mind that many insecticides are cumulative, so that small non-lethal doses over a period of time may build up into a fatal dose. When a well-fed pigeon is starved body fat is metabolised and any stored poisons suddenly enter the system. Acute poisoning results, though the bird has not had recent contact with poison. Some poisons can remain in the tissues for up to three months after ingestion.

Because the insecticides are deposited in fatty tissues, lean birds are more susceptible than fat ones and newly weaned youngsters, or older birds rearing babies in the nest, are more severely affected.

The effect that DDT had on the breeding problems of birds of prey, is common knowledge. Small amounts of poison, accumulated over a long time by the consumption of poisoned rodents, caused serious hatchability problems of raptor eggs, without apparently affecting the parent birds. So serious was the problem that certain species of falcon, especially the peregrine, were practically eradicated from the United Kingdom and elsewhere. Some insecticides were banned and the peregrine falcon was placed on the endangered list and strictly protected by law in an effort to preserve the remnants of the population. In England, these measures have been very successful and the scale has swung strongly in favour of the peregrines.

A constant battle now rages between the protagonists of peregrines, who live almost exclusively on pigeons, and pigeon owners. Pigeon breeders cannot afford to ignore the lesson.

Besides their lethal effect, low doses of insecticides affect the sporting ability of racing pigeons. We know that most poisons are cumulative and have to ask ourselves the following questons;

- How much poison is absorbed by a pigeon following an insectidal dip?

- How long does it take before all traces of poison are eliminated from the tissues of the pigeon?

- When is it safe to dip again?

- Poison is mainly stored in fat. To what extent is the stored poison released when a pigeon races long distances and begins to draw on its reserves of stored fat?

- Would it not be better to not dip at all?

- What would be the effect of repeated dipping on the pigeon's racing performance, remembering that no visible signs of poisoning occur?

- Most important: are the mites and feather lice more harmful than dipping?

I never recommend dipping but would advise the use of powders. If there's any doubt I prefer to live with a few mites and stray feather lice rather than struggle with below-par, poisoned, pigeons.

3. Molluscicides (Snailkillers)

Snailbait is usually produced in pelleted and liquid forms. In the pelleted form, the molluscicides resemble pigeon feed in pellet form, used by some fanciers. Pigeons accustomed to eating pellets, are in danger of being poisoned by snailbait if it is spread in gardens where the birds go foraging.

Trade names include Mesurol, Snailban, Sluggem, etc. and the active ingedients include Metaldehyde and Carbaryl.

Trials done with poisoned pellets have confirmed that pigeons will not die from eating the poison as vomiting is one of the first reactions and before enough of the toxic principal can be absorbed by the birds, the majority is vomited out. If adequate water was taken simultaneously, absorption would be enhanced and more serious poisoning could occur.
   Symptoms include vomiting, incoordination, mis-pecking and haphazard flying. Recovery sets in and is complete in six hours. No treatment needs to be given.

4. Rodenticides

Rodents (rats and mice) are attracted to pigeon lofts because food and shelter is provided at one location. Many rodenticides contain anticoagulants, mainly derivatives of Warfarin (fumarin, choumachlor, difenacoum etc.) and are presented in pelleted form. Warfarin is a relative of coumarin and dicoumarol. Better-known brand names of the rodenticides are Rattex, Finale, Norax etc.

They exert their action by interference with the clotting mechanism of blood, as a result of which, insignificant injuries become major haemorrhagic episodes and death ensues from repeated attaks of internal bleeding. Vitamin K is an effective antidote in all cases that have not progressed to the stage where blood transfusion is required.

Pigeons are relatively resistant to poisoning by Warfarin derivatives. In a small trial, 10g of Rattex fed daily to a pigeon for five days, had no adverse effect. These findings are similar to ones by Garner, who stated that Warfarin is harmless to poultry. The toxic dose of dicumarol for pigeons is $\pm$1g/kg bodyweight. (The toxic dose for the dog being 50 mg/kg)

With the increased familiarity of pigeons to pelleted feed, it is reasonable to assume that a hungry pigeon, if given the opportunity, might partake of large quantities of rat bait. If adverse reactions should occur, injections of vitamin K would be sufficient treatment.

Zinc phosphide, another constituent of some rodenticides, is lethal to all birds and mammals. Gastroenteritis and oedema of the lungs are found at post mortem. Zinc phosphide can be detected from the stomach content in the laboratory.

5. Fertilisers and weedkillers

Fatal poisoning from ingestion of artificial fertilisers or weedkillers has not been encountered. On occasion, fertilisers spread on gardens and lawns, have seriously affected the form and general health, in that racing velocities were below standard and returns were poor.

Case history: Birds were generally unwell, all treatments having been given. On examination the birds were unthrifty and lacking in condition, with scurfy breast skin, bluish in colour – obviously unfit to race. The fielding habits of the pigeons were observed and it was seen that they spent much time in the garden, picking up unknown food. The pigeons were refrained from visiting the garden and their condition improved, losses returned to normal and the fancier's name once more appeared amongst the top placings in his club. The birds had been eating fertiliser, in the form of small grey pellets, that had been loosely spread in the garden.

Weedkillers have become popular with gardeners and though no fatal cases have been noted, they will, when ingested, cause unthriftiness, lack of condition and poor feathering.

As with fertiliser ingestion, the condition is essentially chronic and when the race results are below standard and all other possible causes have been eliminated, one must not neglect to observe the birds outside the loft. Careful enquiries as to the use of fertilisers and herbicides in the vicinity of the loft may provide an answer.

6. Mycotoxins

Mycotoxins are toxic particles produced by bacteria and fungi, which cause disease when ingested or inhaled.

4.1. Ergot

Though not a common cause of disease, ergot poisoning does occur sporadically. Claviceps purpurea, or ergot, infects the flowers of cereal grains, especially rye and wheat, producing mycotoxins. When swallowed, these injure the lining of the vascular capil-

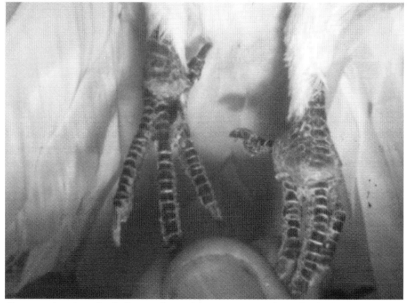

Ergot poisoning, both feet and toes have gangrene from lack of blood supply. Note the inflammation at where the healthy and gangrenous tissues meet.

laries, resulting in restrictions to the bloodflow, which is followed by dry gangrene of the affected parts, usually the toes. If excessive amounts are taken in, the toxin can kill pigeons.

There is no treatment or recovery once gangrene has set in. Such birds, unless they are valuable stock pigeons and not too badly disfigured, are better culled. All contaminated or suspected feed must immediately be removed and destroyed and all feed troughs scrupulously cleaned to remove traces of the toxin.

4.2. Aflatoxin

Produced by the fungus, Aspergillus flavus, aflatoxin has for many years been a problem for farmers and health authorities. All animals are susceptible to aflatoxin poisoning, though poultry and pigeons appear to be more at risk. The fungus multiplies most rapidly when favourable conditions of moisture and heat coincide. These can occur in the growing crop in the field, in the grain silos, in the fancier's grainbin or in unclean feedtroughs.

Peanuts stacked in middens and exposed to rain, followed by a hot spell, have been heavily infected. Fanciers that feed peanuts to their pigeons should have each consignment laboratory tested, to ensure that the nuts are aflatoxin-free, before offering them to their birds.

In recent years large quantities of imported maize were found to be contaminated with aflatoxin and feral pigeons, eating of the corn spilled at shipyard unloading, became ill and died. Apparently the maize crop in the USA had suffered drought, ear rot and insect damage, all of which promote the entry and rapid growth of Aspergillus.

The toxin causes liver damage and lowers the condition of pigeons, resulting in poor race results and increased losses. With liver function below par, failure of proper feed and vitamin/mineral assimilation occurs and the birds become susceptible to other diseases.

The macroscopic autopsy is essentially negative but on microscopic examination of the liver, bileduct proliferation has been seen and is considered almost pathognomonic for the condition. (We found differently, in a small trial performed at our clinic. Mouldy maize kernels, containing 1600 mcg aflotoxin / g maize (obtained from the Medical Research Council), were fed for six days to two pigeons. Autopsy failed to show bileduct proliferation.) We believe that more work needs to be done on the pathogenicity and autopsy changes of aspergillosis toxin for pigeons.

Prevention consists of keeping the pigeons from eating contaminated grain. Aflatoxin on grain can be detected by using an ultra-violet light to screen samples of the feed, which will fluoresce bright yellow if positive, though fluorescence may occur for other reasons. Positive samples must be submitted to a laboratory for chemical and quantitative analysis to confirm the presence of toxin and the degree of contamination. It appears that no trials have been done to determine the level at which aflatoxin consumption becomes pathogenic for pigeons.

Maize, damaged by drought or insects, is more susceptible, as the mould has an easy entry into the kernels. Under favourable conditions (heat and moisture), the moulds rapidly multiply and produce toxin, making the feed unfit for consumption.

To best preserve the maize it must be dried to 13% moisture content as rapidly as possible after harvesting, to inhibit mould growth. Maize with a high moisture content which is stored at high temperatures, is potentially very dangerous for pigeons, as is feed that has become wet and was allowed to remain so.

4.3. Botulism.

Botulism occurs in many animals and birds, but is rare in pigeons. The toxin is produced by the bacteria Clostridium botulinum which organism is usually present in decaying proteinaceous matter, especially meat and carcases.

Pigeons have been known to feed off the maggots that have eaten the toxins in these carcases. The dischages from a dead rodent in a grain store, can be the source of contamination for all of the contents. Some, badly managed, pigeons are avid river bank feeders, where the mud and snails may be contaminated with botulinus toxin. Such foraging birds run a high risk of botulism.

Botulism attacks the nervous system, causing paralysis, which often starts in the neck – hence the term limberneck – progressing to complete paralysis, coma and death.

No specific treatment exists for the condition in birds. Prevention is self-apparent. Pigeons must be in the loft or in the air, never on the ground and never allowed to roam at will. Adequate rodent control is essential for healthy, disease-free pigeons.

7. Salt.

Some fanciers break rock salt into pinhead-sized pieces, which are avidly eaten by pigeons, especially those with babies in the nest. It causes mild chronic nephrosis resulting in loss of condition and reduced racing performance.

Another practice is to feed a small amount of fine-grain salt to pigeons once per week. It appears to do no harm, provided the quantities are not excessive and drinking water is freely available. According to Vogel, 1 to 3 grams of salt daily for one month resulted in an increased water uptake, but no observable pathology. Whether any benefit accrues to the birds is doubtful.

Some pigeon keepers feed salt to their birds by dissolving it in the drinking water. Potentially this is dangerous, particularly if the concentration is high, the salted water is left in the loft for extended periods and no fresh water is available. We see no benefit in feeding additional salt to pigeons, except in standardised multivitamin and mineral additives, which are freely available on a continuing basis.

Salt poisoning can occur in an acute or chronic form. The acute form is seen when salt-starved pigeons, are suddenly given ad lib quantities, with resultant overeating. Severe dehydration and nephrosis occur, with mortalities setting in if water is not freely available. If water is available the excess salt is excreted by the kidneys, resulting in watery droppings.

Symptoms

Symptoms include excessive thirst, respiratory distress, fluid discharge from the beak and leg weakness. Nervous symptoms including depression, excitement, tremors, torticollis inco-ordination and death, were described by Trainer & Karstad.

Autopsy

Lesions seen at autopsy include oedema and haemorrhage, though some autopsies are negative. Microscopic examination demonstrates damage to brain tissue; Oedema, congestion, haemorrhages and cell degeneration with mild perivascular lymphocytic infiltration is seen.

8. Medications

Poisoning with medications occurs when products, beneficial at correct levels, are overdosed or when products are used that are toxic to a species, where the therapeutic level far exceeds the toxic level. The possible poisonings of both kinds are exhaustive and only the commonly-occurring ones will be discussed.

Poisoning associated with species.

All medicines, be they antibiotics, anthelmintics, stimulants or diverse products, require to be administered to certain species in the prescribed way at the prescribed dose. Pigeons are not poultry, nor sheep, nor canaries etc. and there is a wide divergence between different species regarding their response to specific drugs. Eg. We see that mebendazole (anthelmintic – Multispec, Telmin) causes infertility, affects feather growth during the moult, and is generally toxic to pigeons.

Poisoning associated with dosage

Some fanciers fallaciously argue that if one teaspoon of a medicine is good then two must be twice as good. The belief survives because most modern medications are safe at higher than optimum dosages. The reverse is also true, underdosing being practised with the rationale; Because the birds are not very sick (half sick), half the required dose is sufficient. Many medicines, particularly the antibiotics, require a precise dosage to prevent the emergence of resistant strains of germs. Other dangers of under-dosage also occur.

Water uptake

There is a tremendous variation in the amount of water that pigeons drink daily. The normal average uptake (cool winter day) is around 50 ml per day, which can rise to 200 ml or higher under extreme conditions. On cold days the water uptake of resting pigeons drops to below 50 ml per day.

The daily water uptake is increased when:

1. The temperature of the day is high and humidity is low.

2. A high percentage of protein is fed in the diet.

3. Pigeons are rearing nestlings, particularly in the later stages.

4. The pigeons are subjected to strenuous exercise.

When medicating the water of pigeons this must be borne in mind, as overdosing and poisoning readily take place. A strict routine to ensure the correctness of the dose, must be employed.

By allowing 50 ml water (less on cold, rainy days) per pigeon per day, the total amount of water for medication is measured and the correct amount of medicine is added. This is then given to the birds (in a morning and evening dose if desired). When all the medicated water has been drunk (each time), fresh water is put down for the rest of the period.

Alternatively all water put down for the birds is medicated. The total amount of water that the birds will drink that day, is estimated and the full amount of medicine added. Medicated water is then replenished as needed.

8.1. Dimetridazole (Emtryl and others)

Dosage

The dose of Emtryl as supplied by the manufacturer, is 5 g per 8 litres of water, fed for seven days. This dose applies to conditions of moderate climate and exercise, with the birds not expected to drink more that 50 ml water. We concur with this dosage for non-racing birds but when pigeons are actively racing and need medication, a shorter yet effective treatment must be given. We have given 8g (approx. 2 tsp) per 5 litres of water for three days. Longer treatment results in toxicity.

Poisoning symptoms first occur in young birds or birds with babies in the nest.

Symptoms

With poisoning of dimetridazole it appears as if the pigeons have lost their sense of judgement. When attempting to land on a perch, they overfly and crash into the wall behind. This is possibly owing to temporary reduced vision. Swaying from side to side, torticollis and total loss of balance may follow. Loss of condition and occasional mortality sometimes occur.

Result

Withdrawal of the medicine and the administration of Vitamin B complex leads to a rapid and complete recovery. Previously poisoned birds have recovered fully to race successfully and win races.

8.2. Tiamulin

The safety margin for tiamulin (Dynamutilin, Tiamutin) is narrow, three times the recommended dose for three days causing acute mortality in ± 5% of birds. Mortalities were peracute and the first occurred after 48 hours without any prior evidence of malaise. The remaining birds did not exhibit any sign of poisoning.

Autopsy

Severe congestion of all the organs, particularly the kidneys, spleen, liver and intestine was apparent. Haemorrhages were seen in the kidneys, liver and part of the intestine. Leakage of blood into the musculature and tissues surrounding the large vessels was noticed.

Microscopy showed severe congestion of all organs and haemorrhage into the spleen.

8.3. Benzimidazole derivatives

Benzimidazole derivatives (anthelmintics) can cause infertility and feathering abnormalities. Fenbendazole (Panacur) and albendazole (Quadrozole, Valbental, Valbazen) are regularly used by fanciers.

8.4. Vitamin A

Vitamin A deficiency does not occur readily in pigeons hence there is no need to supplement the diet. Normal vitamin A requirements of about 80 to 120 i.u. are usually present in standard rations. Experimentally it has been shown that pigeons are susceptible to excessive doses of vitamin A. When 60 000 i.u. were given daily for three weeks pox-like lesions developed with crust formations on the beak, eyelids and wattles.

8.5. Vitamin B 6 (Pyridoxine)

DeVriese states that Vit. B 6 in excessive doses causes toxicity in pigeons. This occurred when tablets of 100 and 150 mg, formulated for use in humans, were dosed to pigeons, whose daily requirements do not exceed 0.3 mg. Daily requirements are supplied by a standard ration, but if desired, can be supplemented by the addition of Brewer's Yeast, sprinkled over the grains or by feeding fresh greens.

9. Metal poisons

9.1. Copper

Copper Sulphate (CuSO$_4$)

Used originally to control trichomoniasis, copper sulphate has an historical record in pigeon keeping. Used to treat copper deficiency in number of species and applied as a fungicide, molluscicide and footbath, copper sulphate is widely available. Though not readily taken up by pigeons above the toxic level of 0.2% in drinking water, the birds will drink it if no other water is supplied. Pigeons drink from swimming pools, where it is used as an algaecide. Uptake over extended periods will lead to chronic poisoning as copper has a cumulative effect.

An acute outbreak of copper poisoning may be caused by a decrease in the plane of nutrition, fasting, or by severe physical effort (racing). Accumulation of copper in the liver causes liver cell damage with jaundice, bleeding tendencies and kidney damage.

9.2. Lead

Pigeons have suffered lead poisoning when they have eaten lead shot. The pellets remain in the gizzard, from where the lead is slowly given off intoxicating the system.

Treatment for mammals consists of slow intravenous injection of sodium calcium-edetate (Ca EDTA), and could be attempted for pigeons although recurrence would occur if the lead pellets were not removed from the gizzard.

9.3 Mercury

Seed dressed with the mercuric fungicide such as methylmercury dicyandimide is extremely toxic. Pigeons can ingest the seed in their foraging trips or be accidentally fed with the treated seeds. Symptoms may not be apparent for some weeks after the feeding of treated seed has begun. There are no discernible autopsy lesions.

9.4 Zinc Phosphide

Zinc Phosphide, a constituent of some rodenticides, is lethal to all birds and mammals. Gastroenteritis and oedema of the lungs are found at post mortem. Zinc phosphide can be detected from the stomach content in the laboratory.

10. Cyanides

Pigeons racing to the Witwatersrand and Pretoria areas in South Africa, fly over or pass nearby the water pans of the gold mines in Orange Free State and Transvaal. When racing occurs on a hot day, pigeons drink the mine water which is contaminated with cyanides used in the gold extraction process. Mortality usually sets in very quickly.

Poor returns from races may be owing to this poisoning, as positive cyanide poisoning has been diagnosed in returning depressed, moribund racers.

A typical "bitter almond" smell is given off when the stomach is opened. Macroscopically the bright red colour of the blood is noticeable. Laboratory detection of cyanide is possible from the stomach content and from blood but must be done as soon as possible because of the volatility of cyanide.

Treatment for mammals is intravenous injection of 1% sodium nitrite at 25mg/kg, followed by intravenous 25% sodium thiosulphate at 1.25g/kg and may be tried for valuable pigeons.

Chapter 10

Breeding problems

Breeding problems arise with infertility of either the cock or the hen, but determining whether infertility is present, may create difficulties. For our purposes a hen will be reckoned to be infertile if, though all systems are in readiness, she fails to lay normal eggs and the cock will be considered infertile if he does not fertilise the hen's eggs. Both states can be temporary.

These definitions are fraught with potential argument. For example; Is a cock infertile if, with severe arthritis, he cannot mount the hen? Or is a hen infertile because, transferred to a new loft, she will not take a mate? In our hypothetical cases the cock is functionally infertile and for purposes of our discussion, we accept that he is infertile. The hen's breeding cycle is not in readiness, so that she, according to our definition, is not infertile. Because she is not infertile, it does not mean that she is fertile. That first has to be shown – by her producing an egg.

1. Infertility in hens

When the hen can no longer lay and the condition is permanent, she is sterile; if not permanent, she is infertile. Conversely if normal eggs are laid, even should they fail to hatch, the hen is fertile. A hen that lays wind-eggs (eggs without yolk) is considered infertile.

There are a number of reasons for infertility in pigeon hens. They are of varied source and often the etiology can only be surmised, many times the reasons are unknown.

1.1. Age

Old age can end a pigeon's reproductive life although old age is often given the blame when no other reason for the infertility appears obvious. It is questionable whether old age is a cause before the age of 10 years.

Cessation of laying sometimes becomes permanent following a period of irregular laying. Hens first become subfertile, as seen when the period between clutches of eggs is prolonged or when one egg only is laid per clutch for a few months; eventually egg-laying stops. Other hens cease to lay very suddenly.

Certain families continue to lay for a long time, whereas individuals from other families become infertile at a relatively young age but usually not before five or six years.

Treatment

The treatment of infertility in ageing pigeons has erratic results and usually is not successful. Hormone treatment should be the last resort (though it is the first method requested), and is rarely successful.

1.1.1. It is of the utmost importance to get the pigeon into the best possible state of health. Most elderly hens are overweight. This is corrected with diet control and exercise. Where most breeding stock have been prisoners they are allowed freedom and given regular exercise, if possible. Exercise is a primary factor in conditioning the hen.

1.1.2. All birds are given vitamin B complex on a regular basis, i.e. daily or on alternate days. Green feed, deworming, a high protein diet, trace element supplementation and control of erosive diseases like crop canker, coccidiosis and external parasites are essential.

1.1.3. Once the hen has been brought into top physical condition, the cock is brought to her. Ideally they should be locked in a loft compartment on their own, protected from interference by other pigeons. Should eggs be produced one does not want them to be unfertilised because of interference from another cock, nor fertilized by an amorous cock that happened to be nearby and seized a good opportunity. Male pigeons appear to be jealous and will attempt to prevent copulation between a pair, interfering with mating.

Besides the obvious genetic preferences, the choice of mate is not critical and any healthy, fertile cock is adequate. It need not be a young pigeon; an experienced middle-aged lively cock is more suitable. Mating should take place within one or two days and a week later, the cock should be driving if in the company of other pigeons, as driving does not always occur if the pair is totally isolated.

1.1.4. If no mating, calling or driving has begun within the first ten days and no external disturbances are present, the situation needs to be re-examined. Certain questions must be asked.

- Is it the right season? (Some pigeons will breed at any time of the year but starting in early spring through to midsummer, is the ideal time for pigeons to breed, although not necessarily ideal for the fancier.)

- Are there enough daylight hours?

- Are the pair happy with one another? Is either of the pair too dominant? A mismatched pair can do savage damage to each other.

- Are they settled in the loft? If either, cock or hen, is constantly looking to escape, breeding is unlikely.

If no disturbing factors exist, the pair may be psychologically unsuited and the cock exchanged for another.

1.1.5. If there are no eggs two weeks after the pair have accepted each other, the hen is examined. Her vents should be open and relaxed, indicating normal hormonal function. Closed vents indicate that hormone production is inadequate. She must either be given more time to develop naturally or treatment with hormonal injections is begun. Experience in handling eggy pigeons is invaluable, in that some hens will open wide days in advance and others will not open until a few hours before laying.

1.1.6. With the cock driving and the vents open without any indication that eggs are going to be laid, two foster eggs are placed in the nest. The presence of foster eggs will not stop a hen from laying; she will simply add her eggs to the clutch. The cock usually is the first to accept the strange eggs, the hen following 6 to 24 hours later. Going through the motions of brooding and rearing, re-affirms the normal physiological rythm of hormones and helps to finally bring the hen into condition. At no time during the rearing process must the pair be stressed. One nestling is removed if necessary.

At all times there must be an adequate provision of vitamins, minerals, trace elements, shell grit, hard grit and protein. Once the foster babies are about two weeks old, the pair prepare for a new set of eggs.

1.1.7. If the hen again fails to lay, hormonal therapy to promote follicle stimulation is tried. Some success has been achieved but generally the results are disappointing.

Therapy consists of giving gonadorelin (Fertagyl, C.E. Laboratories) which is a synthetic gonadotrophin. Gonadotrophic hormone activates the pituitary, to release F.S.H. and L.H. These induce follicle maturation and ovulation. 0.05 ml Fertagyl is given and repeated every four days till results are seen.

1.2. Disease

Generalised disease can bring about temporary infertility during the acute stages, eg. ornithosis. A prolonged recuperation period and depleted bodily reserves from debilitating conditions, such as endoparasites and malnutrition, can have the same effect.

Localised disease of the reproductive tract can be a follow-on from generalised disease, eg. paratyphoid, or it can arise sporadically from non-infectious origins, eg. abdominal abscess, yolk retention, ovarian tumours etc..

Certain medicines, eg. the nitrofurans, amino-nitrothiazole (Enheptin), dimetridazole (Emtryl) and the benzimidazoles (anthelmintics) have been reported as causing temporary infertility.

To continue the investigation into the infertility of the hen, a physical inspection of the reproductive tract is required. This is accomplished by doing a laparotomy (described in chapter 15) or a laparoscopy. Whatever the outcome of the investigation, the outlook for eventual success remains poor.

Laparoscopy

An otoscope with halogen light source and a longish speculum can be used if a laparoscope is not available. The procedure is performed mainly to sex captivity-bred parrots and other birds. The technique differs little for pigeons. With the pigeon anaesthetized (chapter 13) the scope is introduced into the left abdomen passing through the left abdominal airsac, to view the kidneys, adrenals, ureters, vasa deferens and ovary or testes. Ventral midline entry allows visualisation of the the liver but right-sided entry risks injury to the duodenum. Any bleeding immediately obscures all sight.

Careful examination of the reproductive organs facilitates the etiological diagnosis of infertility.

2. Hatchability failures

Failure of the eggs to hatch is related to infertility of the cock, in which case the eggs were not fertilised, or embryonic mortality which prevents the fertilised eggs from hatching.

For regular development to occur, the egg must be fertilised between 24 and 44 hours prior to laying. After release from the follicle the ovum, which becomes the yolk, normally remains in the oviduct for 41 hours. The first egg is laid 8 to 10 days after coupling.

2.1. Infertility of the Cock

The most common and apparent cause of hatchability failure is infertility of the cock; the eggs have not been fertilised by him. Causes include:

- Old Age

Increasing age results in decreasing effectivity of all systems, including sexual drive and fertility. However, some cocks have been known to produce vigorous youngsters to an advanced age and senility is not the only factor to be considered when the reproductive future of an old cock is discussed. Prolonged fertility is seen in some families or strains, while the opposite is also true, some cocks becoming permanently infertile at 8 or 10 years of age.

As increasing years diminish the physical powers, more care must be taken to preserve the vitality of old stock. When they become arthritic and slow, they are more easily hindered at mating by other cocks. Consequently they should be housed in separate loft sections. Some fanciers find it useful to clip away the vent feathers to facilitate copulation. I am not convinced that it helps but it does no harm and all possible assistance must be given.

Treatment

To treat declining fertility of cocks a similar programme as outlined for hens, discussed previously on page—, is followed. Diet, exercise, health care and general management are all important and the baby rearing exercise is often more successful with cocks.

Hormone therapy aims at improving spermatogenesis and consists of two subcutaneous injections of 200 Units serum gonadotrophin 3 days apart, followed by one injection of chorionic gonadotrophin 3 days later. Additional Vitamin E (alpha tocopherol) is given and results are promising.

- Disease

Any febrile disease can cause temporary infertility. Some specific diseases can directly affect the testicles, particularly paratyphoid, which results in atrophy of the organs and sterility. Pseudotuberculosis, aspergillosis and peritonitis may incidentally cause orchitis with resultant sterility. Treatment in most cases is hopeless but can be attempted for the primary disease condition.

Tumours of the testes are rare. When they occur sterility is inevitable.

- Ambulatory handicaps

Any crippling infirmity will cause functional infertility if it prevents the pigeon from mating successfully. Severe arthritis, gout, tumours of either leg, fractures or similar conditions are responsible.

Cotton or nylon thread entangling a pigeon's toes and not speedily removed, results in gangrene with loss of toes. If an identification ring is too tight, gangrene ensues and the foot may be lost. Such cocks can be functionally infertile and no treatment is possible. Should fertilisation be possible the handicap often results in egg breakages. Physically disabled birds must be in loft compartments alone with their mates.

Malaligned healed leg fractures, resulting in such severe disablement as to make mating impossible, create functional infertility. Fertility can be restored in these cases by correction of the malalignment. This requires rebreaking the malaligned bone, followed by correct setting and fixation, by either internal or external means.

- Medicines

Benzimidazoles (albendazole, mebendazole etc.), 5-nitroimidazoles (metronidazole, dimetridazole, ronidazole and carnidazole), nitro-furans, pyrimethamine and amino-nitrothiazole (enheptine), have all caused problems with fertility. It is recommended that these products are dosed when the eggs have been laid and the pigeons are hatching.

2.2. Overcrowding

Too many cocks in the loft will result in interference with the mating pair. Most cocks will not allow another pair to copulate in their immediate presence, attacking the hen and forcibly jostling the mating cock off his mate. Successful copulation is prevented at the critical time, i.e. between 24 and 44 hours before the egg is laid and if this happens often the eggs are not fertilised.

2.3. Timing

Some hens are fast layers, others are slow. The hens that are quick to lay, i.e. six to seven days after the first introduction, should not be mated to a sluggish cock as he may be slow in mating and unfertilised eggs result. More often the reverse is true. The prelaying period is prolonged to three or four weeks after the first introduction, and the cock, driving for two weeks or more, loses interest and the pair stops mating. Laying at this time results in unfertilised eggs. When prolonged driving exists, it is advisable to break the pair, condition the hen, and to try again some weeks later.

2.4. Early Embryonic Death (Black eggs)

Within 10 days of laying and after candling is positive, fertilised eggs sometimes cease developing and the embryo dies. The timing of embryonic death differs from dead-in-shell, where the eggs are due to hatch but the chicks fail to chip out.
    The causes of early embryonic death include vitamin deficien-cies, chilling, cracked eggs and bacterial contamination.

- Various vitamins affect body growth and a deficiency of some vitamins can lead to embryo mortality. Vitamins essential for normal development within the egg, include vitamins A, B12 (though most is manufactured), B2, B5, B6, E and Folic acid.

Vitamin deficiencies have been thoroughly studied in poultry and do not occur much in pigeons. Results of deficiencies are mainly extrapolated from poultry results.

- Chilling of the eggs occurs when, for various reasons, the parents are forced to leave the nest allowing the eggs to become chilled. Semi-hatched eggs can survive unattended for up to 24 hours, depending on the environmental temperature. Normal squabs are delivered at the end of hatching, though the period is extended for the equivalent time that the eggs were chilled. It should never be automatically assumed that embryos are dead because the eggs were chilled for a time. Especially in the latter stages of incubation, developing squabs are able to withstand a surprising degree of chilling.

Vermin in the loft cause many problems. Apart from transmitting infectious disease, mice create enough disturbance to cause the breeding pigeons to desert the nest, causing chilling. Rats will attack the birds and carry away and eat the eggs.

Overpopulation can be the cause of chilling, cracking and breaking of eggs, through the aggressive behaviour of marauding cocks. The parent, normally the cock, vigorously defends its nest against intruders, and momentarily forgetting the nest, scatters the nesting material and eggs in all directions.

Relative overpopulation with excessive numbers of one sex in the loft, may entice a pigeon away to a new mating, leaving the remaining partner to look after the eggs. Pigeons do not often make good single-parents and the remaining parent soon abandons the nest, leaving the eggs to chill and die.

- Cracked eggs result from insufficient nesting material, disturbances, overpopulation and accidents. The cracked eggshells are liable to become dented or squashed and bacterial penetration of the eggs is increased. Embryo mortality is raised.

A cracked eggshell can be repaired with a strip of adhesive tape (sellotape) and many cracked eggs have delivered healthy young.

- Bacterial contamination on the eggs is increased if the nests are wet, dirty and unhygienic. This usually occurs if the parents have loose bowels or if the nest has inadequate protection from rain. Raised bacterial contamination of the shell, increases bacterial penetration, leading to embryo mortality. Aspergillus, E. coli and Salmonella are the organisms most commonly involved.

Excessive caked dirt on the eggs block the tiny pores in the shell and, if severe, cause oxygen starvation and death of the embryo.

2.5. Dead-in-shell

Chilling, cracked eggs and bacterial contamination, are a major cause of dead-in-shell breeding results. All the various reasons as enumerated above are applicable.

Once bacterial penetration of the shell and eggshell membrane has occurred the bacteria primarily invade and multiply in the protein-rich yolk. Should the squab survive, it often requires help to escape from the egg. It will be somewhat retarded in its development, often with an open navel and poorly absorbed yolk sac. This infected yolk is later drawn into the body where it serves as a constant source of infection, poisoniong the system and preventing healthy growth. Such squeakers never make good racing pigeons and are better culled at birth. The late Belgian champion, Louis Vermeijen, was very strict on this point and never helped a baby out of the egg. Nor did he ever keep a chick that had an imperfectly absorbed yolk at birth.

Paratyphoid is an important and serious cause of dead-in-shell eggs. If management and hygiene are good and dead-in-shell breeding persists, an investigation to rule out the possibility of paratyphoid is carried out. Suspicion is heightened if the dead-in-shell breeding results occur concurrently with severe loss of weight and increased sterility, particularly amongst the breeding hens.

3. Malformed eggs

3.1. Soft-shelled Eggs

Soft-shelled eggs are owing almost exclusively to a lack of calcium in the diet and occur in young and old hens. When it occurs in older hens one must check on the availability of shellgrit (calcium carbonate). In young hens it can sometimes occur with an abundance of grit, probably because the hen has not learnt to eat it. Soft-shelled eggs are also found following sulphonamide therapy.

3.2. Rough-shelled Eggs

Rough-shelled eggs are a lesser version of soft-shelled eggs. They are commonly found in the first round of eggs, particularly if the hen has not been properly prepared.

Rough-shelled eggs occur in infection of the oviduct where the organ is prevented from depositing an adequate layer of calcium carbonate to form the shell. Hens with this problem should be isolated and treated with broadspectrum antibiotics for 10 to 14 days.

Sometimes an ageing hen lays rough- or soft-shelled eggs before eventually ceasing to lay. This indicates degeneration of the genital system and is practically always irreversible.

Certain antibiotics (e.g. Lincospectin) and sulphonamides have caused the formation of rough-shelled eggs. If drugs must be given to breeding stock, it is advisable to administer them in advance of the mating period or immediately after laying, when the hens are brooding.

Rough-shelled eggs are prone to egg-retention, and the possibility of caesarean section is increased.

3.3. Bloody-shelled Eggs

Bloody-shelled eggs occur regularly in young hens under stress. The cause is unknown and the quality of the egg is not affected. First-time layers are more affected and it possibly occurs because the genital system is forced beyond its capacity.

Occasionally a team of birds lay a large percentage of bloody-shelled eggs during the same period. The quality of the youngsters hatched from the eggs, is not affected. The cause is not known.

3.4. Yolkless Eggs.

Some virgin hens produce small eggs, which contain no yolks. Very rarely a hen will continue to lay such 'wind-eggs' in spite of vitamin/mineral adjustment and protein supplementation.

The phenomenon occurs in adult hens at the start of the breeding season if the management during the off season, particularly regarding worm control and protein levels in the diet, was deficient. Upon correction of the relevant managerial lapses, the condition quickly rights itself.

Some old hens lay yolkless eggs when they approach the end of their reproductive lives. Temporary respite may be gained from improved management and diet but the results of such efforts are usually unrewarding.

3.5. Double-yolk Eggs.

As in poultry double yolks occur occasionally in pigeon eggs. I do not know any that have hatched.

3.6. Triple Eggs.

Occasionally a hen lays three eggs per clutch. It is a normal, though rare, occurrence. Pigeons hatched from these eggs are completely normal although it is advisable to rear one chick under foster parents. To require the parents to raise all three, places unnecessary strain upon them and will almost certainly result in all three babies being undernourished and below par.

4. Young chick diseases

Young chick diseases include all conditions affecting young squabs, not exceeding three weeks of age. Most adult diseases affect nestlings and cause mortality, deaths being chronic or acute.

4.1. Chronic Disease

Chronic disease is rare in healthy lofts but can have many causes. Conditions of which the pathogenicity is obscure, are included here.

- It is occasionally caused by a bacterial infection following from incompletely absorbed yolk. The young bird has diarrhoea, becomes dehydated and loses weight. The baby does not seek food as urgently as a healthy nestmate and deteriorates further from lack of nourishment. The parents seem to recognise that a disorder is present and do not make a special effort to provide care. With antibiotic treatment, it may survive but the baby will not grow into a robust, healthy pigeon. Culling is preferable.

- Hexamitiasis can occur amongst the nestlings if the disease is present in the loft. Nestlings from about the tenth day begin to pass loose faeces and deteriorate. The organisms can be recovered from fresh bowel content or from a fresh cloaca smear.

- Adenovirus causes chronic green enteritis toward the end of the nesting period. Some birds may die. Macroscopically, enteritis is seen on post mortem. Histologically, intranuclear inclusion bodies can be found in the liver and intestine.

- Ornithosis occasionally occurs in nestlings. Stress of early weaning promotes the disease in youngsters. Diarrhoea, lack of appetite and wasting occurs. The young birds die or have to be culled.

- Trichomoniasis (crop canker) of the navel is a common disease in Europe. The lesions can spread to the abdominal airsacs. Trichmoniasis of the crop, throat, and liver are seen at an older age.

- Pox lesions can occur on the navel but are relatively seldom seen. Lesions of pox are more commonly seen on the head, wing butts and legs, occurring when mosquitoes abound.

- Polyuria-polydipsia is a common phenomenon in nestlings. It occurs following nephritis and nephrosis, particularly as a result of paramyxovirus.

In the latter half of the nesting stage, polyuria-polydisia sometimes occurs in apparently healthy individuals. The babies pass a copious projectile watery dropping. They are aptly known as "spuiters" in Belgium. No sign of disease is present and both parents are usually healthy. It is surmised that the phenomenon occurs because the parents feed excessive water to the babies. Improvement seen after administration of metronidazole (Emtryl), is thought to occur because the parents, tasting the medicine in the water, reduce their intake and thus regulate the amount of water fed to their offspring.

- Nestlings with rales (gurgling breathing), occurring towards the later stage of the nesting period, show no other sign of illness. The parents also appear healthy. As with the above condition, it is surmised that the symptoms are caused by an excessive amount of water fed by the parents. The babies are unable to swallow the water quickly enough and a small amount enters the trachea, setting up a localised foreign body infection, causing rales. The condition usually disappears spontaneously upon weaning.

- Rickets is seen if calcium grit is not available for the parents. The youngsters are small, depressed with weak bone structure (tested by breaking strength, on autopsy) and often have crooked keels. Culling is best.

Crooked keel can occur where stock is well-fed and the babies are healthy. It is seen particularly where feeding birds are given a large proportion of pelleted feed. The youngsters grow rapidly and muscle development outstrips the calcification process. Besides the crooked keels, no deleterious effects occur and crooked keels are not a detriment to successful racing.

- Coccidiosis is rarely found in nestlings and the significance of their incidental findings, have yet to be clarified.

4.2. Acute Disease

Acute disease is recognised by sudden mortality, no symptoms having been observed. The young birds die in the nest, apparently healthy and with full crops. The nestmate often survives without being affected. It is a relatively rare condition.

- Babies dying from paramyxovirus macroscopically show swelling of the kidneys, some with pale areas. Microscopically interstitial focal nephritis with multifocal parenchymal necrosis of the kidney cells is seen. Infiltration of lymphocytes and some heterophils occurs. The parents may show signs of paramyxo but mortality is rare if breeding is ceased. Birds that continue rearing activities become prone to other diseases and mortalities occur.

- Acute, widespread mortalities occuring in the first three days, oocasionally happen in some lofts. Subsequent breeding rounds are normal and the parents show no sign of disease. Cause is unknown.

- Paratyphoid causes mortality from the fourth day. It occurs in severely affected lofts and other manifestations of the disease are present.

- Ornithosis can cause acute mortality in nestlings. The adult birds usually show signs of the disease.

Chapter 11

Miscellaneous diseases and conditions

A. UROGENITAL SYSTEM

1. Eggbinding.

Eggbinding is diagnosed when the hen cannot pass her egg normally and it is retained in the distal oviduct. If it is the first egg, spontaneous regression of the second developing ovum usually occurs. Dehydration of the oviduct develops in longstanding cases and prolapse of the gravid (egg-holding) oviduct may result.

Experienced fanciers generally have no problem feeling a retained egg in the abdomen. Similar signs are occasionally caused by a tumour or inspissated yolk, and an incorrect conclusion is readily drawn. Where doubt exists, radiography of the abdomen will demonstrate the presence or absence of an egg. Lateral and dorso-ventral views are advisable.

The cause of egg-binding is an abnormal egg, oviduct malfunction or abnormal positioning of a normal egg. Abnormal eggs include double-yolk or rough-shelled eggs. In oviduct abnormality the eggs are normal, as they are when turned sideways, but cannot be passed because of debilitation from calcium deficiency, excessive laying, disease, verminosis or malnutrition.

Oviduct malfunction includes inertia (sluggishness to contract) from calcium deficiency, needed also for eggshell formation and normally withdrawn from the bloodstream and the skeleton. Inadequate dietary replacement affects the nerve network and can lead to reduced oviduct motility, which may be severe enough to cause egg-binding. Paralysis of the legs is occasionally seen just before and during the laying process, i.e. during shell formation, but is of a transient nature.

Mineral supplementation, particularly calcium, during the breeding season is absolutely essential.

Localised conditions of the oviduct, leading to egg binding include inflammmation of the oviduct, yolk retention and adhesions of the oviduct from previous trauma or infection. An inflamed oviduct has reduced peristalsis and reduced capacity for eggshell formation, resulting in rough-shelled eggs, which increases the predisposition for egg-binding.

Treatment depends on how long the condition has been in progress. If of recent origin, the bird is placed in a warm, quiet and dark place and left alone for a few hours. Heat is supplied from a hot water bottle or small electric blanket. Injection of calcium borogluconate (intravenously or intraperitoneally) is usually successful in restarting peristalsis.

Heat and calcium will often resolve the situation. Oxytocin injection (1 – 2 i.u. intramuscular) may be attempted.

Should there be no response to this treatment after about six hours, an attempt is made to deliver the egg manually.

Procedure

A small amount of oil is introduced into the cloaca via a soft rubber tube and spread gently around the egg. This is not easy but greatly facilitates the delivery. With the bird held in the normal horizontal position, one hand is placed over the back with the thumb and index finger resting lightly on either side of the egg, felt through the abdominal wall. The fingers are slowly brought together and the egg is gently squeezed backwards. Great care must be exercised because the pigeon is severely stressed by this manipulation. One should feel the egg moving backwards and if no progress is made, the procedure is discontinued for fear of excessive stress.

Occasionally the egg is half-delivered and covered by the oviduct (partial prolapse), which is stretched to extremes and paper-thin, and into which a small incision is made that greatly facilitates delivery.

Should the above procedure for delivery not be successful, Caesarian section is safer than continued manipulation and must be performed. The operation is described in chapter 15.

The egg must never be broken forcibly. The sharp edges are harmful to the oviduct and damage can result in inflammation and peritonitis. Small bits of shell are difficult to remove and excite localised infection if left behind, frequently leading to sterility and possible fatal peritonitis.

2. Prolapsed oviduct.

Prolapse of the oviduct occasionally occurs during the egg-laying process and may take place at the same time as laying or immediately after the egg has been passed.

When prolapse occurs at the time of laying, the egg is passed enveloped by the paper-thin oviduct, tightly adhering to the shell surface. Immediate action is required to prevent desiccation of the oviduct, which leads to necrosis of the organ and permanent infertility. The life of the pigeon hangs in the balance. A small incision is made in the oviduct through which the egg is released. Subsequent suturing is not required

From this point the two variations are treated similarly. The prolapse is pushed back and a purse-string suture is placed around the vent and left in position for two or three days. With some luck future egg-laying is not affected.

Should the pericloacal tissues be stretched and torn, repeated prolapses will occur. In this case the purse-string suture is left in for ten days, (making sure that defaecation is possible) and the hen is removed from contact with all cocks. She is restrained from egg-laying for three months.

3. Retained yolk

The etiology of yolk retention is uncertain. The ovum is retained in the magnum i.e. the upper section of the reproductive tract and some abnormality in this area, probably infection and inflammation, prevents the yolk from moving down the tract. Excessive layers of albumen are laid down in concentric layers around the ovum but calcium is not deposited. Instead the whole mass becomes inspissated (dry and solid, through loss of fluid) and firmly lodged.

When the yolk is retained, the hen shows all the symptoms of egg-binding or abdominal tumour. Radiography is useful but laparotomy is the only method that conclusively provides a diagnosis. (On radiology it is difficult to distinguish between inspissation and tumour.) The inspissated mass almost fills the abdomen causing respiratory distress and the hen shows an open, rounded epiglottis and pendulous abdomen.

The operative procedure to remove the yolk consists of laparotomy, followed by an incision into the large irregular oviduct and piecemeal removal of the inspissated mass. The procedure is relatively easy but time-consuming and very stressful to the bird. It is essential that all the little bits of material which adhere to the oviduct wall are removed. A few interrupted sutures hold the edges of the oviduct incision in apposition and the abdomen is closed following standard procedures.

The success rate of the operation is low, as extensive degenerative changes have occurred in the genital tract and these hens must be regarded as infertile. The procedure is reserved for special cases and a guarded prognosis is always given.

4. Sex Reversal

An apparent change of sex (pseudohermaphroditism) sometimes occurs in pigeons, as it does in other birds. The conditiuon must be differentiated from hereditary hermaphroditism (presence of functional male and female organs in the same animal), which was described in a family of pigeons by Riddle. In this family, 80 % of the cocks had a left ovotestis with oviduct and oocytes, plus a right testis with accessory structures. True hermaphrodites are otherwise rare.

Pseudohermaphroditism (sex reversal, sex change) is relatively common and is responsible for the male characteristics developing in a hen. Tumours, hormonal imbalance, infection etc., produce a new level of hormones that cause the body to override the existing secondary sexual characteristics. Artificially this condition can be produced by testosterone injection.

Grades of sex reversal is seen. When in the extreme, pseudohermaphroditism occurs, and true hens (egg-laying) change to cock-like individuals, capable of fertilisation. In nearly all cases the situation involves a hen, apparently reverting to a cock, although correction of the status (apparent cock back to hen) does occur.

5. Nephrosis

A severe fatal proliferative interstitial nephrosis, apparently infectious, has been seen on a few occasions. The birds sicken over a period of a few days to a week. Hens appear to be more susceptible. Signs of gout are prominent prior to death, which occurs before the bird looks very ill. The etiology is unknown but a viral or toxic origin is suspected. All outbreaks to date have spontaneously regressed with about 10% mortality.

On post mortem examination the kidneys are excessively enlarged and bulge from their bony crypts. They have a solid consistency, glistening appearance and greyish-cream colour. The remainder of the carcase appears normal.

No treatment appears to be effective, although protein restriction in the diet was useful for minimising the severity of the gout attacks. Uric acid, which accumulates subcutaneously in the legs, exudes from a cut made in the skin.

B. MUSCULOSKELETAL SYSTEM.
6. Leg weakness

Two syndromes occur.

6.1. During the summer months particularly, some pigeons are presented with an acute disability to walk normally. The bird waddles a few paces, then lies down on its sternum. The condition mainly occurs amongst adult pigeons and stock cocks appear to be more susceptible.

It would appear as if the condition is more painful than paralytic. The legs feel warm and the bird seems unwilling, more than unable, to walk. The condition improves following a few days of antibiotic medication, the choice of which does not appear to be important, making it doubtful whether antibiotic therapy is necessary. Spontaneous recovery does occur. Sick pigeons are removed from the loft to prevent their being savaged by marauding cocks and to allow them time to eat and drink.

Autopsy examination has revealed small whitish/grey spots distributed through the muscle groups (paratyphoid?), without other changes found in the rest of the body.

6.2. Calcium deficiency is a definite and common cause of paresis in hens either just prior to, during, or after laying. The calcium necessary for eggshell production is derived from the blood stream and skeletal system and if not replaced by dietary intake, insufficient circulating calcium results in impaired nerve function to the muscles, giving rise to paresis of the legs.

Treatment, using a subcutaneous injection of calcium effects a quick response but the provision of shell grit or some other form of easily-digestible calcium (eg. cal-C-vita), is essential for continued good health.

7. Muscle Binding

Muscle binding in pigeons is seen when the normally supple breast muscles become turgid, hard and very swollen. The birds are unable to fly or fly very poorly.

Some experience is required to recognise this condition and novice fanciers may be fooled into thinking that the bird is in top-form, 'blown' with condition and in good shape to win a difficult race. Nothing could be further from the truth. If sent to a race in this condition the bird would probably be lost.

When forced to circle, affected birds go up reluctantly and drop onto surrounding roofs, treetops or the ground, a few minutes later. At times the condition is mild and difficult to recognise and even experienced handlers are deceived. If doubt exists the pigeon should be held back to race on another day. Any pigeon that suddenly and for no apparent reason, develops extraordinary 'condition' must be viewed with suspicion.

The etiology is unknown. It may occur in the flock or in separate individuals. It would appear that over-exercise followed by rest, plays a role. We have seen it also following the usage of certain medicines e.g. furazolidone. It appears to be a metobolic condition but more research is needed to clear up the puzzle.

Treatment is effective. A mild purge, with Epsom Salts ($MgSO_4$) and Bicarbonate of Soda ($NaHCO_3$) mixed in equal amounts and given at a dosage of 1 teaspoon per litre, is followed by multivitamins in the drinking water. Light feeding (high ratio of clipped barley) and rest, with no exercise for a few days, resolves the problem. There are no after-effects .

8. Foot lesions

8.1. Bumblefoot.

Bumblefoot is diagnosed when the metatarsal pad of the foot becomes infected and swollen. It is usually not a flock problem, occurring in individual birds only. The condition is caused by a secondary infection, following trauma to the pad (eg. puncture by foreign bodies). Numerous organisms have been isolated from the lesions, of which Staph. aureus and E.coli are the most common.

Treatment of bumblefoot requires surgical excision, debridement and lavage. This is best performed under light general anaesthesia. A tourniquet is placed distally on the leg to limit haemorrhage, which may otherwise be extensive. Adequate bandaging and antibiotics, locally and systemically, are indicated and continued with until healing has occurred. During the recuperation period, the bird is housed in a cage with a clean smooth floor.

8.2. Foot pad ulcers.

Foot pad ulcers are found in individual birds and the condition probably have a similar etiology to bumblefoot. Repeated trauma on a hard rough floor is the main cause and healing occurs only if the floor is suitable. Regular applications of a disinfectant ointment such as povidone iodine, improves recovery. If no response is obtained to local treatment, the ulcers may be excised and healthy tissue sutured in place. Control of haemmorhage, antibiotics and post operative bandaging are essential.

8.3. Hyperkeratosis

In this condition the footpads produce excessive horny tissue which grows to a considerable length and thickness (nearly always bilateral). Lemahieu has found a genetic factor to be involved. Some fanciers claim that cement floors are etiological.

Excessive horn is cut away from time to time and a light oil applied to soften the hard, horny tissue. Resection of the pads has been recommended (as for bumblefoot) but if the condition is extensive this would not be practical. Hyperkeratosis is not dangerous and may be left untouched. It seems to worry the owner more than the pigeon.

8.4. Gangrene & necrosis

Dry gangrene of one or more toes is occasionally seen. The toes become dark brown to black, undergo necrosis, dry up and eventually fall off. Although the dead toes do not worry the pigeon, live tissue at the interface with necrosed parts is swollen, inflamed and tender. If many toes are affected and large areas are necrotic, the pigeon may show signs of generalised illness. The etiology has not been identified but is thought to be the ingestion of seed, contaminated with ergot (a fungus growing on cereals).

Treatment is reserved for valuable breeding birds. The necrotic toes are amputated through the viable section, sutured and bandaged. Bleeding is profuse and must be controlled. Antibiotics and bandaging are mandatory. If enough of the stump remains the pigeon may lead a normal breeding life, especially if the defect is unilateral.

Metal identification rings may become too narrow for birds with strong bone development, resulting in reduced blood flow, swelling and necrosis of the foot. If seen in time the ring may be removed and the leg and foot saved. Narrow, short-beaked scissors are used to cut the constricting ring. The ring can also be sawn through with a fine metal saw. Great care must be employed to prevent damage to the swollen leg and foot during the procedure.

If the leg is lost at about the level of the ring, breeding becomes more difficult. Breeding cocks with only one foot must be isolated and protected from other cocks, to ensure successful filling of the eggs. Amputated hens and cocks tend to break eggs if disturbed, so that separation from other pigeons is advisable. Their eggs are placed under foster parents whenever practical.

Cotton thread

Many feral pigeons lose toes and sometimes a foot when they become entangled with cotton or nylon threads. As time progresses, the thread which was originally loosely draped around the toes is pulled tighter, causing swelling and eventually necrosis. A pigeon's toes easily become entangled and it is imperative that all threads, especially plastic and nylon, are removed from the vicinity of the pigeon loft.

9. Spread legs

The abnormality is seen uni- or bilaterally in young babies still in the nest. It is usually discovered at the feathering stage or later, and is caused when the nest is constructed with insufficient nesting material. Nestlings whose nest is built on a smooth surface are particularly vulnerable. The condition occurs more frequently when only one baby is raised per nest, as the slip-stop provided by the second nestling is absent. Nests situated on a very shallow space, encouraging the birds to kick out the nesting material, are prone to rearing youngsters with spread legs.

Anatomically there is a abduction and outward rotation of the leg, from the hip to the hock with the femur rotated 10°, the knee (femoro-tibial joint) 15-20° and the tibia 60-80° normal. Eventually the foot is 90° and more, rotated. In cases older than 10 days, the bones and joint have "set" and the condition is irreversible. Young-sters intended for racing, are best culled. In early cases, treatment is accomplished by preventing abaxial positioning of the legs with tape, fixing the legs in the normal position.

The legs of a valuable squeaker intended for stock, can be made more functional by means of an operation, once the bones have completed their growth and hardened. Fracturing, reverse turning and internal fixation is involved. See chapter 15 for the details.

10. Wing disease

There are many causes of wing lameness but the term dates back to 30 or more years ago, when 'wing disease' was a common problem. From what we can establish it probably was a form of paratyphoid – where the wing joint(s) became inflamed, swollen and eventually semi-mobile with the bird flying in a lopsided fashion. Once affected these pigeons were permanently crippled and finished as racers.

10.1. Paratyphoid is today still seen occasionally. It is the most common pigeon disease in Europe and introductions should be carefully screened. See chapter 5 for a detailed discussion of the disease.

10.2. Accidents are a common cause of wing lameness. Particularly on windy days pigeons are prone to colliding with telephone wires, tree branches, fence wiring and even motor vehicles. Serious damage can be caused to the wings, breastbones, legs etc. and many unrecognised internal injuries occur. Injured wings are easy to spot as they hang limp, are often swollen and the feathers are disturbed or stained with blood.

Any pigeon that inexplicably returns late from a training flight or race, must be carefully examined for collision injuries. Often the damage is minor (internal?) but it must be noted and treated, thus preventing valuable birds from being sent to races in an unfit condition.

When bone fractures (humerus or radius-ulna) occur, the bird is usually discarded for further racing – as the wing invariably does not recover well enough for the bird to race again successfully.

However, a fracture of the forearm is not hopeless if either the radius or the ulna is intact and can provide stability for the frac-tured bone. Acting as a natural splint, it prevents serious displace-

ment and further injury. Cage rest for four weeks, followed by
light exercise, can lead to full recovery. We have witnessed a
pigeon, that had fractured his ulna the year before, win a race
from 250 miles (400 km).

10.3 Paramyxovirus affects mainly the central nervous and
urogenital systems, but occasionally the peripheral nervous
system is affected, particularly the nerves to the wings. Acute
severe paresis or paralysis results, leaving the pigeons lopsided in
flight or unable to fly. No other discernible pathology is found
when these birds are clinically examined.

10.4. Pigeons with acute mild wing lameness, the cause of which is
not certain, are regularly seen. When present in a loft, three or
more cases are often afflicted within a few weeks, suggesting an
infectious origin. Nothing may be noticed in the resting state,
depending on the severity, but in flight the birds are slightly off-
balance, with reduced wing movement on the injured side.
    Clinical examination often reveals nothing. Sometimes it would
appear as if the area of the shoulder joint is slightly swollen.
Concurrent with the wing problem, the pigeon tends to lose condition, although it is not clear whether this caused by pain, resulting
in decreased food uptake, or whether it is part of the disease
process. Serum testing for salmonella antibodies has been negative.
    Careful examination on sectioning the pigeon, usually reveals a
negative picture. A yellow gelatinous exudate has, on occasion,
been found to occur in the tissues surrounding the shoulder joint
suggesting trauma. Histopathology of the tissues has not revealed
any specific disease. More case material is needed, with full histo-
ries and clinical examinations, before an etiology can be found.

11. Gout

Gout is a metabolic disorder, characterised by the deposition of
uric acid and urates in various parts of the body, in place of excretion via the kidneys as is normal. In the pigeon two forms of the
disease are recognised, namely synovial and visceral gout,
depending on where the metobolites are laid down.
    Visceral gout is extremely rare. The condition usually occurs
when some or other serious disorder of the kidney is present,
inhibiting normal metabolic function. Gout has been seen in the
absence of observable renal disease, indicating that complex mech-

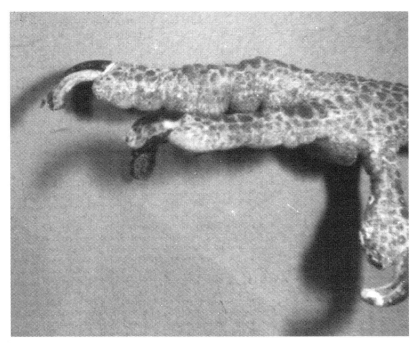

Synovial gout, white urate crystal accumulation in the tendon sheaths is visible through the skin.

anisms are involved. More research is necessary before the condition can be adequately explained.

Visceral gout is seen only on autopsy, the pigeon usually having died very acutely and the condition appears as a thin white deposit of urates evenly spread over the internal organs, especially the heart and liver.

Synovial gout occurs more readily, is very painful for the bird and the process is largely irreversible as the urate crystals once deposited are not readily reabsorbed. The urates are deposited around the tendons and joints and are visible through the overlying skin as focal pale areas. When the skin is incised the white pasty fluid oozes out.

C. DIGESTIVE SYSTEM

12. Sourcrop

Sourcrop is a widely-used term given to a variety of conditions affecting the crop. In the terminology of the racing pigeon fancy, it includes all forms of crop malfunction as these mostly result in a sour-smelling crop content, whence the name originates. Conditions leading to sourcrop include: candidiasis, overfilling with food and water owing to obstruction, enteritis, poisoning, bacterial inflammation and physiological retention with souring of pigeon milk such as rearing parents restrained from feeding young.

A watery crop content, resembling pendulous crop, is noticeable with birds suffering from acute enteritis.

Non-specific crop infection results in an overfilled watery crop, which results in delayed crop emptying. Rapid improvement is achieved with manual emptying, antibiotic dosing and restriction of water intake for a few days.

Candidiasis, the classical sourcrop, is rarely seen, but is diagnosed on culturing Candida albicans from the crop fluid. Treatment is by giving Mycostatin (nystatin), 0.5 ml twice daily. Full discussion in Chapter 5.

13. Yellow liver disease

At autopsy we occasionally recognise a condition that we have provisionally termed 'yellow liver disease'. It is a serious and important cause for the failure of pigeons to race satisfactorily. The birds appear well except that they fail to gain condition normally. Some may show some loss of appetite and train somewhat lethargically but appear otherwise well. With careful nursing, which consists mainly of rest, selective training and good feeding, they put on some condition only to break down after a training flight of 45 to 60 minutes.

Having excluded all other possibilities autopsy is performed and reveals a severely pale, slightly atrophied liver, without other significant changes. Histology has not to date revealed any significant pathology. Blood enzyme studies have not been adequately experimented with.

The condition appears suddenly but the extent of spread of the disease, throughout the loft, remains unknown, as identification of affected birds in the live state, is not yet possible. Laparoscopy would provide an answer but is impractical. At autopsy, up to 100% of cases have been seen in some lofts out of five or six investigated.

The colour of an affected liver varies according to the degree of the condition, appearing initially as pale streaks, which coalesce as the disease progresses, to form an overall pale ochre-yellow liver.

Proper preparation for racing is impossible. Birds are carefully nurtured to preserve their physical condition and are forced to forego road training. The effect on racing is devastating. The birds manage to return home when race conditions are favourable but on hard days or at long distances up to 100% losses have been recorded.

14. Enteritis

Some forms of enteritis not described elsewhere under specific etiologies, are discussed.

14.1. Ulcerative enteritis of pigeons

With some tongue-in-cheek this disease has already been included under the virus diseases in Chapter 2. Justification is found in the classical virus-like behaviour of the condition and appearance of the microscopical lesions.

The disease is highly contagious, as was evident in 1985, when in a period of six weeks the condition spread across a zone of 60 miles (100 km), affecting hundreds of lofts from independent organisations with different transporters. The disease is self-limiting and occurs in birds of all ages but youngsters are more susceptible.

The symptoms are those of enteritis, with loose droppings of mushy consistency and severe loss of condition, followed by gradual recovery. When the ulcers perforate, aspergillosis and airsacculitis become a problem. Airsacculitis causes thickening of the airsacs, leaving the bird useless for racing, though it may be used as a breeder.

Autopsy typically reveals ulcers in the intestine, sometimes throughout its length but more usually confined to the distal bowel for a distance of about 10 to 20 centimetres. The lesions may be seen from the outside of the bowel as small raised areas on the serosa. On the mucosal surface typical crater-like ulcers, about 4 to 5 mm in diameter, are found. The bowel is slightly thickened. Bacterial cultures have been negative for pathogens, except in one case where a pathogenic E. coli was isolated.

Histology of diseased bowel tissue reveals intranuclear inclusion bodies – confirming the suspicion of viral etiology.

Treatment with various antibiotics did not make much differ-ence, although chloramphenicol appeared to reduce the severity of the condition – probably due to the control of secondary invaders. More work is be needed to be able to identify the pathogen.

14.2 Acute haemorrhagic enteritis

Occasionally a peracute, haemorrhagic enteritis occurs, affecting pigeons of all ages. The first signs of an outbreak, are when dead birds are found in the loft. Mortalities are limited to a single outbreak resulting in the acute death of two or three birds, or the disease may linger, in which case sick birds are regularly seen, deteriorating till death occurs.

Autopsy reveals cyanosis and a toxic appearance of the carcase. All the organs are dark, hyperaemic and purplish/red in colour. The intestine is filled with a watery, dark brown to red fluid and the wall of the bowel is dark red, paper-thin and flacid with prominent but thin bloodvessels. The mucosa is red and sloughs easily.

The cause of the condition is unknown. Poisoning has been strongly suspected, as the birds have very often been foraging prior to the outbreaks. Unfortunately, when only one or two birds die, the incident is usually not brought to veterinary notice and valuable information regarding the etiology of the condition is lost.

15. Foreign body disease

On rare occasions, pigeons usually hens, swallow metal objects such as nails or bits of wire. The reason for this behaviour is obscure. Some birds are found having swallowed as many as eight nails. The nail or wire passes through the crop to the gizzard where it remains, while the muscular organ attempts to grind it to paste. However, the strong contractions only succeed in pushing the offending nail through the wall of the gizzard and into the abdominal cavity, where it sets up a severe and often fatal peritonitis.

Symptoms shown by such a bird include inappetence and loss of weight, while remaining active and bright-eyed. It eats little and the droppings are poorly digested, some times containing bits of food, or whole grains. Eventually the bird dies from starvation.

Treatment. Radiographic examination will confirm whether the condition is present, following which corrective surgery may be performed. We have had a hen laying eggs less than four weeks after a steel nail was removed from the gizzard. Fortunately she did produce winners subsequently, so the exercise was productive, for us as well as the owner. The operative procedure is described in chapter 15.

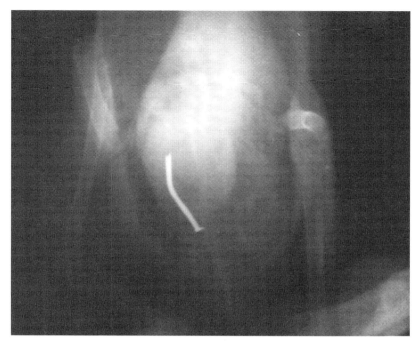

X-ray photograph of a pigeon pierced by a nail. In this case the nail protrudes backwards from the gizzard and is readily operable.

When the birds are kept on short rations and are excessively hungry, it occasionally happens that a pigeon swallows a large piece of maize husk, which has not been not removed from the grain mixture. Husk that swells in the crop and is too large to pass into the gizzard, can be palpated in the crop and physically removed during a minor operation. Husk which passes to the gizzard remains there, posing a more serious problem. Symptoms are similar to when a nail has been swallowed. In addition, repeated swallowing attempts are seen and the pigeon appears stressed. Weight loss is rapid and death occurs within ten days.

D. CARDIOVASCULAR SYSTEM
15. Ruptured Aorta

Very rarely an apparently healthy pigeon, sitting quietly on his perch, suddenly falls off and dies, or falls dead out of the sky whilst flying.

On autopsy, the aorta is ruptured close to the heart and the peri-cardial sac is filled with blood. Death is owing to acute cardiac failure from the inability of the heart to expand normally in the blood-filled pericarium. The rest of the carcase is normal.

The condition is usually seen in birds younger than one year. The cause is unknown. Copper deficiency in turkeys causes a similar condition – whether this is comparable in pigeons is unknown.

Some authorities believe that erosive trichomoniasis, affecting the large bloodvessel walls, is the cause of the rupture.

E. RESPIRATORY SYSTEM.

17. Ammonia fumes

Because of the practice of deep litter on loft floors, we are occasion-ally presented with ammonia fume irritation in pigeons. The condition occurs when the fancier has allowed the deep litter to get wet, or if the birds have had loose droppings, eg. with enteritis. If normal pigeon droppings do not dry sufficiently, are allowed to accumulate under perches they give off ammonia fumes. This happens particularly in rainy weather and at a time of high atmo-pheric humidity.

Overcrowding and poor loft ventilation compound the problem, which is presented as an irritation of the upper respiratory system of the birds. They have wet eyes, red throats and sneeze continu-ously. They are severely stressed by lack of fresh air and are susceptible to secondary infections, particularly aerocystitis caused E. coli and Aspergillus fumigatus.

18. Ruptured airsacs

Ruptured airsacs present a puzzling situation to the first time observer. The pigeon appears blown up like a balloon, over its entire body but particularly in the region of the neck and head. When held in the hand the typical soft airfilled spaces under the skin are felt. If pressure is applied a sharp crackling sound is heard. The condition arises when an airsac ruptures, either from trauma or a disease process.

Treatment consists of puncturing the skin and manually pushing out or sucking out the subcutaneous air with a large syringe.

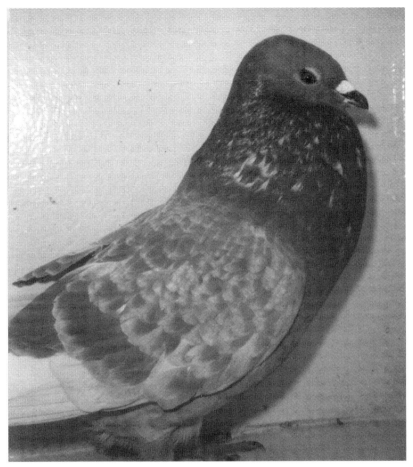

Ruptured air sacs have resulted in air accumulating under the skin, especially in the head and neck

Following removal of the air the bird is confined to a small cage to restrict its movement. Antibiotics are administered routinely to prevent infected airsac complications.

Most pigeons with the condition make an apparently uneventful recovery but few go on to become successful racers. The airsacs are an integral part of the respiratory apparatus and must be in perfect order for racing. It appears that these birds have sufficient resident airsac damage to preclude success at racing but they may be used with great distinction for breeding.

F. INTEGUMENTARY SYSTEM.

19. Abnormalities acquired during feather development

19.1. Nutritional deficiencies.

Composition of the diet has a marked effect on moulting and feather growth. This was superbly illustrated by protein diet studies done on house sparrows. The birds were kept on iso-caloric diets with differing amounts of protein. During the course of the trial the bodyweights of the birds remained constant, but the moult was significantly affected. In birds on a 3% protein diet, moulting was reduced in intensity and time, while birds on 5% protein, moulted on an intermediate level and those on 9% protein, had a normal extensive moult.

We have observed similar effects in pigeons. It must be remembered that these findings apply not only to adult moulting birds but also and especially to babies growing their first set of feathers. Already protein-hungry because of the rapidly growing muscle tissue, a deficiency at this time has a serious effect on feather production. Arginine appears to be the most important amino acid for feather growth. Hemp (whre legal), flax (linseed) and sesame seeds are good sources of arginine.

Not much is known (as yet) about specific nutritional deficiencies as possible causes of feathering abnormalities in pigeons. In poultry a number of such abnormalities have been recorded and it may be assumed that similar deficiencies would lead to similar defects in pigeons.

Niacine and panthothenic acid deficiencies may cause a lack of small feather development. Lysine deficiency causes decreased pigmentation while a shortage of methionine has been found to cause loss of feathers in an otherwise normal skin. Deficiency of arginine and zinc in growing chickens causes breaking off of feathers, blood quills and depigmentation. In addition, leg deformities occur in chickens on a zinc-deficient diet.

Overall protein deficiency causes poor growth, poor feathering, blood quills and pipey feathers. Because their requirements for protein, vitamins and minerals are generally higher, feather abnormalities are seen in young growing birds, more so than in adult stock.

19. 2. Frets.

Frets or hunger lines are seen in feathers that have developed a
break across the beards and quill – caused by severe stress and
lack of food over a short period of time. When a growing feather is
totally deprived of adequate nutrition for a few days, it stops
growing for that period and when fully grown the feather is
marked by a hunger line.

The condition is encountered when growing babies are not fed for
a few days or if a racing bird, moulting a pair of primaries, has a
very hard race and stays out a few days. Often a hard long
distance race of the previous year is reflected as a hunger line on a
primary in the following year. The fret in pigeons is similar to a
break-in-the-wool seen in sheep following a serious febrile condition.

19. 3. Pipey feathers and blood quills.

Instead of unfurling normally, a new soft feather may remain

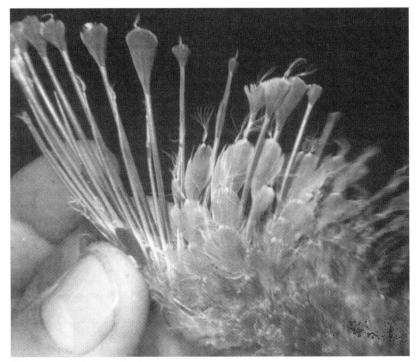

Severe case of pipey feathers.

encased in its sheath for an extended period. This is known as pipey feather. Usually the sheath is sloughed off at a later stage and an apparently normal feather remains.

Blood quills are feathers where the quill, especially the lower section, remains blood-filled for an extended period. The main shaft has a dark purple appearance and bleeds profusely if traumatized. Blood quills are usually also piped to a certain extent. Small feathers also may be affected, and may remain as blood-filled needle-like shafts.

We believe that interruption of an adequate dietary intake, resulting in a subsequent delayed growth of the plumage, be it new feathers or moulted, is the basic cause. A disease condition of the baby or the parents, or improper management for a few weeks can be responsible. Recently we have seen pipey feathering of the neck plumage as result of an excessive concentration of sodium hypochlorite (eg Milton) in the drinking water. Retarded moult was caused.

Mature flights, that at one stage were pipey feathers or blood quills, are the first to shown signs of wear and tear when subjected

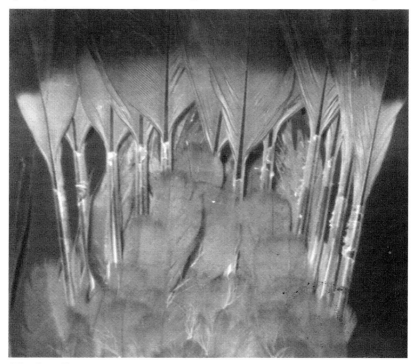

Blood quills.

to the stress of hard racing. It reflects that all was not well in the growing process.

Should pipey feathers or blood quills be present in youngsters in a severe degree, they must be culled; it is better breed new healthy babies – from egg to adult.

19. 4. Pinholes.

Pinholes are pinpoint holes found at random in the vanes of the feather, usually arranged in short irregular rows. Though often encountered, their etiology remains controversial. Dovecote pigeons have numerous pinholes but in well-managed lofts they are absent.

Some authorities claim that the common pigeon louse, Menopon latum, cause pinholes. Others have suggested that the free-living feather-eating moth, found wherever feathers are allowed to accumulate, might be responsible. We believe that the pigeon fly, Pseudolynchia canariensis, is the sole cause. We have seen a correlation between pinholes and the presence of pigeon flies too often, to ignore the derived conclusion that they were caused by Pseudolynchia, in the growing stage of the feather.

We have yet to see a loft where pigeon flies were present during the feather-growing stage and where pinholes are absent. Conversely, when a loft did not have pigeon flies during the moulting period, there are no pinholes. In their search for blood, pigeon flies attack the rolled-up blood-filled young quills, which only display the damage caused by the bites when they unfurl.

There is no treatment for the damaged feathers. If the damage occurs on a subsidiary primary or secondary flight, we extract it and allow a new healthy flight to replace it. Though their effect is not serious, we dislike seeing pinholes, as their presence is a reflection on the management.

As the pigeon fly is a carrier of pseudomalaria, the presence of pinholes leads to an examination for Haemoproteus columbae, the causative organism. A blood film is examined under oil magnification (1000 x) for the parasites. Pseudomalaria interferes with successful racing.

19. 5. Medication.

Various medications have been incriminated for causing feather abnormalities and care must be taken with the use of any drugs, the effects of which are not fully known.

Some deworming remedies eg. the benzimidazoles, are capable of causing severe feather aberrations by their deleterious effect on developing feathers. In the moulting season, fenbendazole (Panacur) and mebendazole (Mebenvet, Telmin) have caused falling out and weakening of feathers, even when used at the recommended dosages.

When the often-used sulphonamides (e.g. sulphamezathine), is given to stock birds with 10 to 12-day old babies in the nest, depigmentation of the growing flights of the young birds, may result. Potentiated sulphonamides (eg. Whitsyn S – sulfaquinoxaline + pyrimethamine) cause depigmentation of growing flights.

Corticosteroids can cause feathering abnormalities.

Antibiotics in overdose (e.g. Tylan), have had severely detrimental effects on pigeons – so much so that a season's crop youngsters have had to be destroyed.

19. 6. Virus Infections

Any severe infection of short duration, causes a break in growing feathers and produces 'hunger lines'. Certain virus infections may cause specific feather defects.

Paramyxovirus infection interrups the growth of feathers, which resume growing after about a week, some of the shafts having formed a weak section and the vane not having grown. A clear demarcation thus forms between the new and previous growth, resulting in the feather being 'pinched' at this point. The new section grows to full length, with the older part forming a 'flag' at the tip. The 'flag' usually drops off but some neck feathers retain the 'flag', creating an untidy appearance. When the 'flag' has been lost, the tip of the remaining feather looks tattered, having lost its original design. The phenomenon can occur following other conditions, and apppears even when no signs of disease hace been observed.

19. 7. Feather stunting.

Feather stunting occurs when the follicles are damaged, the feathers forming with the same defects annually. The etiology of the condition is unknown. Genetic factors have been mooted as a cause, though breeding trials with affected pigeons, produced normally-feathered youngsters. More research is needed before the etiology can be clarified.

Paramyxovirus is occasionally responsible for severe stunting of feather growth.

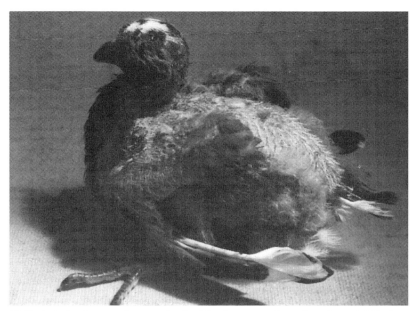

Follicle infection resulting in lack of feather growth in the affected follicles.

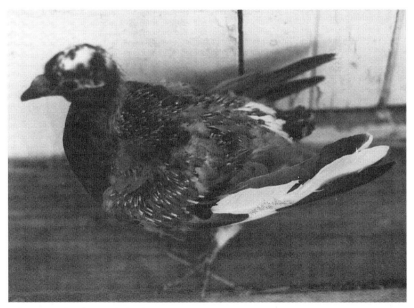

The same bird seen left after the infection has been treated and new feathers are growing from the follicles previously affected.

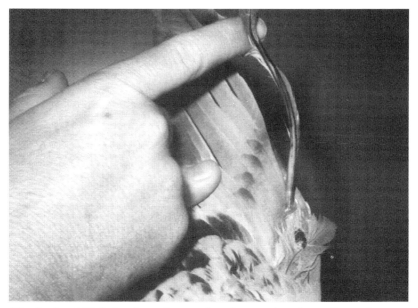

The feather follicle has been damaged and extracting the malformed feather will result in a further distorted feather replacing it.

19. 8. Split Quills

The proximal thicker section of the shaft, usually of all the bigger primary flights, is split down the centre, usually for a distance of one to three centimetres. The part of the feather which attaches to the body is intact and splitting starts usually about two centimetres from the proximal end (calamus). Split quills are believed to be of genetic origin and careful breeding can successfully eradicate the condition.

19. 9. Malformed flights.

Twisted or otherwise malformed flights result from follicular damage following trauma or infection. Rarely the pigeon shows an abnormal feather amongst its baby feathers in which case the condition could be hereditary. Follicular damage is permanent and when malformed feathers are moulted, they regrow with the same abnormality.

Extraction of a malshaped flight results in regrowth of a duplicate misshapen feather. Minor deformity of a flight does not preclude successful racing and races have been won with birds that have had lesser flight abnormalities. When the abnormal flight interferes with racing, the deformed section is removed and replaced with the equivalent part, cut from a normal flight, in a procedure which is similar to fixing a broken flight. A description appears on page 214.

As the condition is not hereditary, an affected bird produces offspring with normal feathering.

20. Abnormalities acquired after moulting

20 1. Breast patch.

A breast patch is seen when a variable number of the small feathers in front of the neck, are frayed and broken, forming a bare patch. Usually the same birds are affected every year.

Ectoparasites were originally thought to be the cause but it is now commonly believed that mechanical factors are involved. The pigeon displays while eating, inflating his clavicular airsacs. At first this causes fraying of the neck feathers, which later break off to leave a bare breast patch. The problem is readily solved by placing a platform on which the bird must stand when eating or drinking and by smoothing the edges of the food and water bowls. The patch will remain till the bird has moulted and if the eating and drinking arrangements have been effectively changed, breast patches will no longer be seen in ensuing years.

20. 2. Soiling by oil.

Occasionally birds return from a race soiled by oil which has leaked from the transporter. If it is light diesel-type fuel, nothing needs to be done, other than to provide adequate bathing opportunities. Within ten days all signs of soiling will have vanished.

Soiling by heavy crude oil, such as occurs when seabirds are caught up in an oilslick on water, occurs rarely. When it does happen, as when lost birds return weeks after a race, the affected pigeon must be washed in dishwashing detergent. Time must be allowed for the body to replace the natural oil and powder, which is removed by the washing.

20. 3. Broken flights

When a primary flight breaks at any time during the racing season, one of three procedures may be followed.

20.3.1. If the tip of a flight is lost, racing is not affected and the flight feather is left undisturbed.

20.3.2. If the damage is such that racing is affected, we prefer to extract the flight, allowing a new one to replace it. The time factor is important. If the damage occurs immediately prior to an important race, we leave the flight, fixing it and extract it later, if necessary. The smaller primary flights take only two to three weeks to grow back, whereas the bigger flights, such as numbers 9 or 10, take six weeks to regrow.

20.3.2. It would be disastrous to a pigeon's winning chances to extract a major flight two weeks before a big race. A number 10 primary, dropped or pulled a few days before an important race, or dropped in the pannier en route to the race point, does not exclude the bird's winning chances. The lack of a flight is not painful, but a soft young number 10 flight, four to five centimetres long and filled with blood, is uncomfortable and easily injured during a long and hard race, being on the leading edge and bearing major stress.

Repair of a flight is readily achieved. Using a very sharp blade the extremity of the broken feather stump is cut in a V-shape. A flight of the same number from a like-sided wing, is cut in a chisel shape to dovetail with the prepared stump. (Experienced fanciers keep left and right-sided flights in store for such an emergency.) Careful attention is paid to the length of the replacement part so that the repaired feather is equal in length to its opposite number in the other wing. A light sliver of wood with high tensile strength, such as a from good toothpick, is shaped to fit inside the hollow shaft. Half of it is glued, fitted into the distal replacement part and allowed to dry, following which the other half is glued and sunk into the proximal stump. The splint should slide into each feather end for about 2 centimetres. Proper alignment is ensured to prevent rotation of the fitted part. If carefully performed the repair work will last until the feather is moulted out.

20. 4. Bent flight feathers

When examining the wings of our racers, we often see a flight that has been bent and stands at 30 degrees or so from the normal axis. The flight is repaired by holding the damaged part of the feather over a steaming kettle spout for a few seconds. The procedure is completely painless and accomplished within 20 seconds, depending on the severity of the damage. The bent quill straightens itself and 30 seconds later, no sign of damage is discernible. For interest's sake, a moulted flight feather may be taken, thoroughly crumpled and held over steam for thirty seconds. The effect is remarkable.

20. 5. Premature feather wear

White feathers have less wear resistance than coloured ones. If any pigeon has an excess of white in its plumage, especially the primary flights, this may lead to excessive wear, fraying of the flight ends and reduced performance. No treatment is possible but the phenomenon must be kept in mind when planning the matings for the next season. Cocks and hens that produce excessive white plumage in their youngsters should not be mated together.

A different type of premature wear occurs if the birds were on a protein-deficient diet during the moulting season. Fraying occurs in the webbing of the flights and can be seen as dark dull patches before wear damage becomes obvious. Attention to correct the diet is necessary to prevent the problem in future stock.

20. 6. Failure to moult

Moulting is a normal physiological process and, dependent on the circumstances, occurs during a predetermined period each year. Stress, from a variety of causes, interferes with the normal cycle, interrupting it entirely or in part. The main stress factors in pigeons are disease, continuous hard racing (and training) and excessive breeding, particularly if accompanied by poor nutrition. These factors cause the moult to be retarded and some feathers, not moulted timeously, may be retained for the ensuing year.

Occasionally we see a pigeon that fails to moult one or more of its primary flights. The bird will not have been sick and in all other respects the moult will have proceded without incident. This frequently is the result of damage to the follicle, either from injury or localised infection and the feather often regrows normally after extraction. If examined carefully, the proximal end of such an extracted flight may be seen to be covered with dry blood or inspissated pus, indicative of the condition which prevented extrusion of the feather. Having removed the diseased feather the follicle can recover and resume normal follicular function. Future moults run a normal course.

G. GENETIC and CONGENITAL ABNORMALITIES

Pigeons produce relatively large numbers of offspring annually and this, coupled with the generalised practice of inbreeding followed by outcrossing, produces many genetic variations ....including pigeons with extraordinary racing potential, which is the ultimate aim of the racing pigeon breeder.

Unfortunately these practices also work in reverse and produce genetic variations that are abnormal – being so severe that they are sometimes unable to fly. Consider the many and varied shapes, sizes and colours found amongst the fancy pigeon varieties, where each breed was selected for some or other anatomical variation and how, by selective breeding, the effect of the variations was increased through succeeding generations to modern times, where some of these birds are barely able to fly. Remember that all pigeon breeds, including racing pigeons, were derived from a common source, the wild pigeon, Columba livia.

When undesirable variations are recognised in racing pigeons, most racing fanciers suppress the babies at an early age and consequently very few are presented for documentation. Scanty records of genetic abnormalities are therefore found in the pigeon literature.

We have come across a few abnormalities and present them for interests' sake and also hopefully to stimulate more pigeon people to record the odd variation that they might breed. When the variations do not affect the racing ability of the pigeons they are retained and some of these birds have become famous racers.

21. Genetic and Congenital Variations that do not Interfere with Racing

21.1. Crested Head.

Feathers growing retrograde on the back of the head and neck to form a crest pattern. Inherited as a simple recessive character. Some very famous racers and breeders have had this abnormality.

21.2. Frill.

Similar to crest (see 21.1). Inherited as a recessive character, not simple – possibly partly sex-linked. Seen as a patch of feathers growing haphazardly and wrong-way-round on the front of the neck stretching to the chest. Theoretically it might affect flight by interference with the streamlining of the pigeon and if severe cause enough of a burden to make successful racing difficult. Successful racers have had frills.

21.3. Feathered legs.

Inherited in a partially dominant fashion. Though mild feathering is not disadvantageous it is not advisable to mate pigeons with feathered legs with each other. Besides the added burden of carrying the extra mass of the leg feathers, severe feathering causes the ordinary metal identification rings to become too small, cutting off circulation and promoting gangrene. When the ring is removed, as it must to preserve the foot, the pigeon becomes useless for racing.

21.4. Eleven flighters.

This interesting peculiarity is seen in certain families but it is doubtful that there is an advantage for racing. If there had been, the phenomenon would be common in our winners and champions. Selective breeding has established families of eleven-flighted birds and such families regularly produce pigeons with 11 flights bilaterally and occasionally some with 12 flights.

Theoretically if one wing has eleven flights and the other has ten, there should be some imbalance, with disturbance of smooth flight. There is no evidence to support this, as unilateral eleven-flighted birds have managed to become good winning racers, though not in greater numbers, relatively.

21.5. Webbed and extra toes.

Webbed toes are seen fairly regularly, extra toes are rare. Because most fanciers do not like seeing the web, which is usually found between the middle and outside toes, it is slit through when the youngster is a few days old. The foot develops normally and there is no hindrance to racing.

Hollander's research into webfoot, revealed that the condition has a worldwide spread with an equal distribution between the sexes. He found that some web-footed birds were winners at 500 and 930 miles (800 and 1500 km).

Birds are seen with extra toes: known as polydactyly. Both webfoot and polydactyly are inherited as recessive to normal.

At routine post mortem, we found intra-abdominal feathers in a web-footed pigeon. It is not clear whether there is any correlation between web foot and internal feathers but the latter would be a source of foreign body irritation and predispose the pigeon to infection. Such a pigeon would not race successfully.

21.6. Feather colour variations

Colours vary widely and mutations are occasionally seen. Amongst these are mosaic i.e. a bird with different colour plumage eg. as red on one side and blue on the other. Mosaic colouring does not affect racing and mosaic pigeons have been known to breed winners.

22. Genetic and Congenital Variations that interfere with racing

22.1. Fancy breeds.

Most variations found in the many breeds of fancy pigeons, are detrimental to flying, as the characters were not selected for

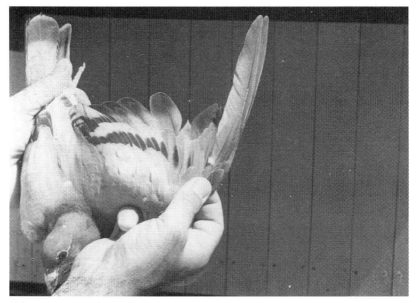

Permanent abnormal feathering, each year's feather growth will repeat similar defects.

racing. Some breeds can fly well, eg. the tippler, but it will never win a good race, neither will a tumbler, a pouter, a fantail or a meat producer like the Gross Mondaine. Through mutations and selective breeding for different qualities, some of these varieties have difficulty flying at all.

22.2. Extra wings.

We have seen one specimen bred from normal parents, with an extra pair of wings. It was probably a mutation and as such would

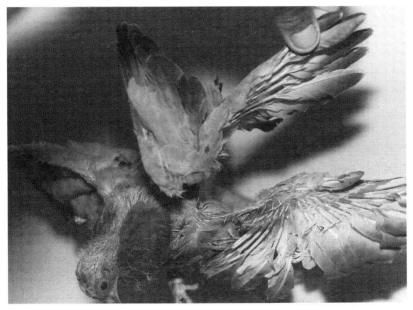

A four-winged pigeon, thankfully a very rare genetic problem.

have been capable of reproducing its own kind. In the racing world such obviously incapable pigeons are usually destroyed early in life.

22.3. Silky.

When in the homozygous state these birds are incapable of flight, as their feathers have lost binding capacity. Heterozygous birds are attractive curly-feathered specimens, capable of limited flight.

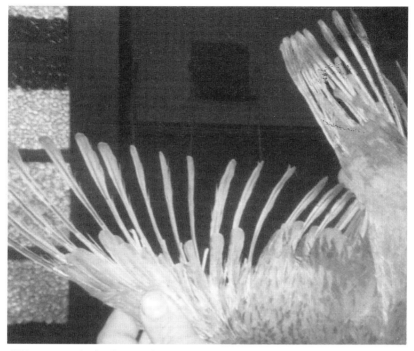

Silky, a genetic feathering fault.

22.4. Micropothalmia.

Severely deficient eye development make these pigeons unfit for racing.

22.5. Double feathers.

Cases are on record where birds developed an extra set of flight feathers – fitted to the same wing. Little is known of the cause and possible genetic constitution of such cases.

Extra tail feathers attached on the lower back just anterior to the normal tail, have been described. Birds such as these are more of scientific interest than practical value and are usually destroyed early in life, before breeding trials can be done to determine their genetic make-up.

22.6. Lethal genes.

A large variety of lethal genes have been described in various species particularly in mammals and they undoubtedly occur in pigeons. In pigeons however, many affected chicks die in-shell, making recognition and further investigation difficult. As far as we are aware, no work has been done on this in pigeons and the field awaits the energy and enthusiasm of a keen reseacher.

H. GENERAL
23. Heat Regulation

The maintenance of a stable body temperature requires a constant balance between heat production and heat loss. The heat-regulatory system in the pigeon is very efficient and pigeons have been known to thrive in hot (not humid) conditions. Heat loss occurs mainly from the skin (via conduction and convection) and from the surfaces of the lungs and airsacs (mainly via evaporation and convection).

High environmental temperature and humidity, restrict heat loss and at the critical body temperature, extra heat loss can be regulated only by increased evaporation (increased rate of respiration). Reduction of heat generated is seen when pigeons are forced to fly on hot days. The wing stroke is reduced in volume and output is at a minimum. Races on hot days have relatively low velocities because of a minimal energy production by the pigeons. The wing beat does not travel the full distance, from above the back to below the chest, but is more akin to gliding. The wing moves a short distance above and below the horizontal, keeping energy production at a minimum.

Heat Stroke

The increase in evaporation is inversely proportional to the relative humidity of the environmental air. Ambient humidity thus assumes a major role in the heat-regulatory process.

When too many pigeons are kept in a confined space (too many birds in a training pannier with insufficient ventilation eg. the boot of a car), high environmental humidity and temperature result. Pigeons suffer heat stroke when they are unable to increase their temperature loss and the body temperature rises above the upper critical level.

Before the pathological degrees of heat stroke are reached, stress on the birds gradually increases. Though no symptoms of heat stroke occur, birds that are stressed like this on a regular basis, will fail to develop top form.

The symptoms of heat stroke include vomiting, imbalance, inability to stand or fly, droopiness, weakness and death.

The autopsy is mostly negative, with dehydration and nephrosis as main change. The kidneys are swollen and pale.

Treatment consists of cooling the body as quickly as possible; cold water baths or showers are best. The water must be in contact with the bloodvessels on the underside of the wings. In valuable pigeons isotonic NaCl (Sodium chloride – common salt) with 5% glucose can be given subcutaneously.

• TRAUMA AND SURGERY •

Chapter 12

General considerations

Although the general principles that apply to surgery on mammals are applicable, special considerations warrant discussion.

Incisions, sutures and healing

When incising the skin, haemorrhage is avoided wherever possible by steering away from the vicinity of the larger feather follicles, particularly if the feathers are not fully grown. Some authors advocate tearing the skin but we do not find this necessary, preferring to use straight sharp/blunt scissors for all skin incisions. In muscle tissue we use a blunt dissection technique as much as possible. Hyfrecation of bleeding vessels is effective but stress-producing and is avoided when possible.

Pigeons do not readily absorb catgut sutures and it is preferable to use non-absorbable monofilament suture material. Suture material that is readily digested by pigeon tissue, would be ideal. Further research in this field is required.

Pus formation

Birds do not have lysozymes in their white blood cells with the result that pus and blood become inspissated, coagulating and forming solid lumps within the tissues and body cavities. This is beneficial, insofar as pus does not spread readily to other areas, helping to localise an infection and the pus is not easily absorbed, effectively preventing septicaemia.

The penalty suffered for this convenience is that pus and blood-clots are separated from normal tissue but remain trapped within the body – unless there is some opening through which the unwanted material can be extruded. This has far-reaching effects. When the edges of a contaminated wound are sutured, the blood and pus which intervenes between the healing edges effectively prevent cohesion. The wound needs to be cleaned before adhesion can begin. If sutures are holding inspissated matter within the wound edges, manual removal of the cheesy material is necessary before the wound can heal.

Bandages

Sutured wounds are usually left uncovered. Bandages are difficult to apply snugly and pigeons do not readily tolerate them or leave them alone. Being accustomed to regular preening of their feathers, they attempt to remove anything that, to them, represents unwanted material and dirt. However pigeons endure such material better than other birds.

Restrictive bandages around the body are sometimes useful with wing fractures. Legs often have to have protective bandages. Socks and slings are occasionally used when multiple leg fractures are set.

Pain and Stress

It is erroneous to assume that pigeons feel pain sensations similarly to mammals. Although difficult to judge and almost impossible to measure, it seems that pigeons respond differently to certain stimuli that would be painful to mammals.

Birds seem to experience no pain with incisions and pigeons respond little to small operations, which can consequently be done without anaesthesia. They appear relatively unconcerned about a broken leg. They respond quite sharply however, to feather extraction and pressure, especially on the legs, toes, joints and tendons. Joint and tendon inflammations are extremely painful (e.g. paratyphoid or gout), and the limbs may tremble with pain. Very often, when birds are thought be paretic or paralysed, they are in fact fully mobile but prefer to rest on the breastbone because of pain experienced in the legs.

Pigeons are relatively resistant to shock. Pain does not appear to cause severe shock and pigeons (as opposed to some other birds) are quite resistant to sudden drops in temperature. They are, however, very susceptible to shock caused by dehydration and may die acutely, if deprived of water when suffering from severe nephritis or enteritis. When healthy and in good condition, a resting pigeon can live without food or water for four to five days, showing little outward appearance of distress.

Pigeons are able to withstand increased environmental temperature fairly well, reducing their daily exercise to a level commensurate with their ability to deal with the heated air. Beyond a certain level, however, they cannot compensate. The increased respiratory rate effects cooling by increased evaporation. When the humidity of the environmental air is increased, this cannot occur and the pigeon's ability to accomodate to an increase of temperature in humid conitions is severely limited. Pigeons enclosed in a training pannier, cardboard box or boot of a car are at risk if adequate ventilation is not provided.

Conditions bringing about a reduction of the airflow, cause respiratory embarassment, which creates severe stress in pigeons. They include:

- compression of the respiratory apparatus, whether it be external eg. by being held too firmly in the hands or internal eg. by a large space-occupying body in the abdomen.

- compression of the trachea, eg. conditions and injuries of the neck.

- diseases that narrow the lumen of the trachea, eg. granulomatous tracheitis, ornithosis, pigeon herpesvirus.

In cases of respiratory embarassment, mortality occurs before the stage is reached where one might have expected the pigeon to die. This happens particularly if the stress on the birds is increased e.g. by forcing them to fly, creating shock conditions that lead to death.

Chapter 13

Anaesthesia

No easily-administered anaesthetic agent has yet been found that gives persistently good, safe and effective, general anaesthesia in pigeons. Although ketamine (Ketalar) in combination with xylazine (Rompun), is widely used and generally gives good results, some violent and unpredictable periods of excitability, are experienced.

Local anaesthesia

Local anaesthesia does not give good results in pigeons. Adequate infiltration to reach desired levels of analgesia, may result in acute intoxication because the anaesthetic dosage relative to bodyweight is too high.

General Anaesthesia

Three to four hours of pre-anaesthetic fasting is desirable. Ketamine, in combination with Xylazine, is generally used. It is essential that surgical instruments and equipment are in readiness, as the required depth of anaesthesia is quickly reached. Anaesthesia usually lasts approximately 30 minutes and wherever possible, prolongation of anaesthesia must be avoided.
   An operable depth of anaesthesia is judged to have been reached when;

- the toe reflex is absent,
- the cornea reflex is slowed,
- the respiratory rate drops back to normal or slightly below,
- total muscle relaxation is present.

Inhalation anaesthesia is used in small species of birds but is less successful in pigeons. Halothane, methoxyflurane and ether have all been used with success but have complications. Volatile anaesthetics require intubation for succcessful administration.

Halothane 2-4 % may be administered with oxygen and mixed with nitrous oxide (50/50) (enhances analgesia and reduces the amount of halothane given).

Methoxyfluorane is safe but at 4% provides insufficient analgesia for most procedures.

Alphaxalone with alphadolone (Saffan) can be used for ultra short-acting anaesthesia at a dose of 5-7 mg/kg bodyweight. Anaesthsia lasts 5-7 minutes.

We use $\pm$20 to 35mg ketamine (Ketalar) with 3mg xylazine ($\pm$0.1ml Rompun – Bayer AH) given i.m. in an average pigeon (350 g -500 g). There is a rapid action (three to five minutes) which lasts 30 minutes or longer and care must be taken not to start the operation before the pigeon is fully anaesthetised. The bird will lie down very quickly (two to four minutes) and appear so flaccid that one is tempted to ignore the checks for depth of anaesthesia, resulting in spasmodic wing beats at inopportune times. Should the pigeon require more anaesthesia (either to deepen or lengthen the state), further injections may be given. This usually has the effect of extensively lengthening the recovery phase, and great care must be taken with "topping-up" dosages.

Chapter 14

Pre- and post-operative care

Preparation

Pigeons are generally more resistant to wound infections than mammals but standard aseptic techniques must nonethelesss be employed before, during and after surgery. Preparation of the operative field is restricted to the essential area, as plucking of the feathers over a large area is painful and stress-producing.

While holding the skin, one or two feathers at a time are carefully removed by plucking gently in the line of growth. Very often a tweezer or forceps is best used for the purpose. If a handful of feathers is grasped and pulled the skin may tear – and probably will! – especially in the region of the crop or neck. This is particularly true when an open laceration is present.

Having plucked all the feathers immediately surrounding the operative site, the remaining feathers are soaked in a liquid soap. This effectively wets and plasters them down and out of the way. It traps loose fluff and scales, which would otherwise contaminate the surgical site. An iodine solution, applied to the skin a few minutes before surgery begins, completes preparation of the site.

Haemostasis at wound-closing is meticulously applied because blood clots, trapped between opposing skin edges prevent a wound from healing. They remain in position until extruded by the body or manually removed. If blood oozes from the skin while suturing, the skin is juxtaposed in a few places only, leaving large sections through which dead blood clots may be extruded. Sutures remain in place until blood clots between the edges have been removed, and the wound has healed satisfactorily.

Post-operative care

Suture sites are sprayed with a commercial antibiotic-containing plastic skin and covered with a very fine layer of cotton wool. When dry, this adheres to the skin, forming an effective protectant layer, well accepted by pigeons. Sutures are usually removed 10 days post-operatively, at which time any inspissated pus or dried blood clots are removed from the wound. The sutures situated where clots were present, are left in place for another 10 days, when the process is repeated.

Nursing care following an operation is very important, particularly during the anaesthetic recovery phase. Heat is essential, as anaesthetised stressed pigeons easily become hypothermic and lack of heat markedly prolongs recovery time. We find a small electric blanket with a three-level heat control very handy and use it routinely for all birds post-operatively. It is also very effective when pigeons become egg-bound and often prevents the necessity for surgical intervention.

Care must be taken not to apply excessive heat, as the pigeons are usually confined to a small recovery box or basket which heats up very quickly.

Antibiotics are given pre-operatively and continued post-operatively for four days or until healing is complete.

Chapter 15

Surgical conditions and their treatment

1. Tumours

External neoplasms are removed according to standard surgical principles. They are usually easy to excise and because they are seldom malignant, the effort is well rewarded. Unfortunately many fanciers leave the tumours to grow until their size makes them inoperable.

Special attention is given to removal of growths in the neck area. The skin of the neck is loose and elastic and it is easy to bring the wound edges together after excising a relatively large growth, leaving little tension in the wound. However the oesophagus of the pigeon is extremely thin-walled and has weak peristalsis. A slight pressure, caused by post-operative tension owing to the lack of skin, results in obstructive constriction, leading to starvation and death. When lack of healthy skin occurs, the wound edges are closed as much as possible without creating tension in the skin. An open wound with a patent oesphagus is preferable to a closed wound and constricted oesophagus.

Other skin is not so freely available and before operations are performed elsewhere, one must first estimate whether sufficient healthy skin remains to cover the excised area.

Internal neoplasms, in contrast, are often malignant. Because their owners are frequently unaware of their existence, the pigeons are brought in for attention with the growths in an advanced stage. Often an egg-laying problem is suspected. Some growths, particularly cancers of the ovary, are easy to remove but invariably regrowth occurs within a few weeks.

Abdominal Operation

A transverse or lateral abdominal incision is made, approximately one centimetre away from the breast bone. By carefully pushing aside the intestines, the growth can be viewed. The growths often are friable and likely to bleed, but with careful manipulation they can be exteriorised, tied off and removed. The pigeon can withstand an advanced degree of surgical trauma, before shock sets in.

Excess fat, forming intra-abdominally in some hens during the winter months, may interfere with egg-laying and need removal. This is easily accomplished but it bears remembering that the condition may be genetically transmitted, in which case one would not wish to perpetuate the specific gene combination.

2. Abscesses and blood clots

Abscesses and bloodclots, found in subcutaneous, intramuscular or intra-abdominal sites, may require surgery. A small incision with curettage may be adequate treatment for simple subcutaneous abscesses. Anaesthesia is not necessary. Post-operative antibiotics are advisable.

Intramuscular, multi-layered yellow-brown irregular masses which break up upon traction, are blood clots intermingled with inspissated pus. These lumps of cheesy matter may invade deeply between the muscle layers, effectively preventing healing. Occasionally a sliver of wood or other foreign body, is found wedged into the fibres of the injured tissue. Foreign materials are easily removed and healing is rapid.

Following crash accidents (when a pigeon flies into a window, wire, motor car etc.) internal bleeding may occur from a ruptured liver or other internal organ and large blood clots collect intra-abdominally. Laparoscopy will confirm the diagnosis. If unattended, they remain for prolonged periods causing general malaise and respiratory distress. Following successful removal, healing is rapid and uneventful.

Abscesses consist of crumbly cheesy material, usually encapsulated and easy to remove without damage to the surrounding tissue. Subcutaneous abscesses are found in paratyphoid infection and all abscesses of doubtful origin require to be cultured for the presence of salmonellas. Following a positive test result, treatment, vaccination and culling of carriers must follow.

3. Beak abnormalities

3.1. Scissor beak.

Upper or lower beak deviations to either side, creating a scissors effect, is not uncommon. Some are caused by injury or diseases such as pigeon pox, but in many instances the etiology remains obscure. Should the abnormality cause eating problems, the beak is clipped. Hyfrecation does not stop the bleeding, which may be profuse. Shaping of the beak is repeated regularly, as the beak persists with abnormal growth and unless the pigeon is very valuable it is better destroyed.

3.2. Split beak.

Occasionally, usually in young birds, one sees a separation at the tip of the mandibles (split symphysis), caused by trauma. Drilling a hole from side to side and fixation with soft stainless steel wire, may be attempted. Old injuries have a guarded prognosis, but fresh ones recover well.

3.3. Swallowed maxillae (upper beak).

Trauma is responsible for this rare condition where the upper beak is bent ventrally at 90° and forced into the gullet. It occurs in young birds under four months of age when the beak is still soft and pliable. When first seen it would appear as if the pigeon had lost its upper beak. The bird is not unduly distressed and while forcing the mouth open, the maxillae is lifted out of the throat. The beak straightens itself and returns to normal. No lasting aftereffects are seen.

3.3. Parrot mouth.

Parrot mouth occurs as a result of damage to the upper beak, upsetting its growth pattern, which results in uncontrolled cell division and beak growth. The maxillae grow in a downward curve and the mandibles (lower beak), maintaining a close apposition wiith the maxillae, follow the direction of growth. The damage arises from physical trauma or from infection, especially with pox virus. As long as the bird is able to eat well, the condition is not serious. Should eating become difficult, the beak must be trimmed at regular intervals as the condition is permanent. If eating is not affected it is preferable not to interfere.

4. Nail abnormalities

Nails grow to abnormal lengths in some pigeons and have to be trimmed periodically. It appears to occur in certain families and genetic factors are suspected. Clipping is easily accomplished with ordinary nail scissors provided one does not trim too short, in which case profuse bleeding results and electric cauterisation becomes necessary.

5. Crop and Skin injuries

Skin injuries are bruises, abrasions or lacerations and usually result from collision with wires, tree branches, TV aerials etc. and attacks from birds of prey. The injuries can be mild to extremely severe and occur especially when the birds are flying in strong wind. If pigeons must fly under strong gusty wind conditions, the smaller the flock the less likelihood of their crashing into dangerous objects. Lacerations occur mostly in the neck, crop, breast and leg areas. Raptor attacks cause lacerations mainly on the back, neck and wings.

Rupture of the crop is not unusual. Pigeons with a torn crop eat and drink normally but water leaks from the injured crop. Injuries may be very severe, with water flowing from the torn crop as rapidly as the bird drinks it. Severe injuries often have food stuck to the edges of the wound. Pigeons are surprisingly shock-resistant following such injuries and make an uneventful recovery in a short time. At times a crop injury is initially not observed and only when water dribbles from the it, is the laceration noticed.

Many a pigeon fancier has borrowed needle and thread, to suture an injured bird. Pigeons heal very well and very severe crop rupture can be repaired. Cotton sutures can be left in the skin as they will eventually disintegrate. It is preferable to suture the crop and skin individually.

Small skin wounds are best cleaned and left open. Interfering feathers are gently pulled out. Clipping the feathers around the tear is effective, but once the wound has healed it leaves an unsightly clipped area, which remains until the next moulting period. The wound heals rapidly, with minimal scar tissue formation and proper feather alignment.

When larger lacerations occur, the wound edges are gently plucked clean, the skin is dabbed with an iodine solution and debrided (dead blood and devitalised tissue is removed). Pigeon wounds usually are not contaminated with sand and other extraneous matter but are soiled by disrupted feathers, blood and mangled tissue. Old dry blood, firmly adherent to the tissues (muscle usually), is left undisturbed, and covered with skin, leaving an opening, through which old blood and pus can later be extruded. The skin is closed with a simple interrupted sutures of non-absorbable material (nylon, cotton or silk). Antibiotic plastic skin is sprayed onto the damaged area to help prevent post-operative wound infection. External sutures are removed after ten days.

In severe cases with extensive areas of bleeding, bruised and devitalised tissue, it is sometimes advantageous to proceed in two stages. Once debridement has been accomplished, the skin edges are brought together and sutured with simple interrupted stitches but only in a few places, leaving open gaps between the sutures. Ten days later, the bird is again taken in hand and all blood clots, inspissated pus and devitalised tissue which prevent wound healing, are removed through the gaps. Healing is in process and necrotic material, which has separated from the live tissue, can be removed and the clean edges sutured. If necessary the process is again repeated 10 days later.

When the skin is stripped away from the underlying tissue over a large area, leaving it uncovered, immediate attention is required. It usually occurs in the breast area. The wound must cleaned and covered as soon as possible, to prevent dessication of the exposed tissues. If surgery cannot be performed immediately, a few temporary sutures are placed to hold the skin over the injured area until more precise surgery can be performed.

6. Fractures

Following collision with telephone or electricity wires, television antennas, branches or similar objects, fractures are common and often occur simultaneously with skin damage and trauma elsewhere. Leg fractures can be repaired successfully, but serious fractures of the wing seldom heal without some permanent loss of mobility. Many different techniques have been described and employed, to set fractures of the leg.

Provided two basic principles are observed, the results of most fracture repair techniques are excellent:

- The splint must fit the injured part snugly and provide maximum stability to the fracture.

- The broken leg or wing must be set in the most functional position.

Care is exercised to prevent the external splint from being applied too tightly. Bad technique in applying a splint, can lead to swelling of the foot with possible necrosis. If seen in time the pressure is relieved by removing the cast or splint, which is replaced as soon as the swelling has subsided.

We will examine a few methods, concentrating on those techniques which has given us consistently the best results.

6.1. Toe fractures.

Fractures of the toe are rare. They are splinted with a match-thick sliver of wood approximately 2 cm long, which is taped to the toe, if needs be in the company of the neighbouring toe and is removed after two weeks. It forms an effective, low-cost splint.

Toe fractures can be left undisturbed and will heal without treatment. The pigeon is preferably kept in isolation for two weeks. Crooked healing of a toe following fracture, does not affect racing and is not serious.

Anterior toes must be prevented from bending backwards and special care is taken to stop the pigeon from walking on a bent toe. After ten days the bent position has become fixed, and correction requires difficult corrective physiotherapy.

6.2. Metatarsal fractures.

The metatarsus is the ring-bearing part of the leg. Relatively easy to splint when broken in the centre of the shaft, it can be complicated to set a fracture that occurs under the ring, near the foot or near the hock.

A fracture in the central area of the metatarsal bone is best immobilised in a gypsona cast. Standard gypsona (plaster) bandage, cut into strips ±3 cm. x 10 cm. are folded lengthways, to make the strips easier to handle when wet. With the leg in traction and the fracture reduced the soaked strips are wound around the leg, from just above the hock joint down to the foot, shaping the plaster closely to the leg.

A wood-and-tape splint, as used for tibial fractures, can be used successfully on metatarsal fractures.

When the fracture occurs near the hock joint, the plaster must incorporate the joint and extend halfway up the tibia. The leg is fixed in about 60° flexion. It is less comfortable for the pigeon and becomes quite weighty. Accurate reduction is difficult to maintain when applying the cast.

When the fracture occurs near the foot, the foot is included in the cast. Two lengths of aluminimum wire, one posterior (behind) and one anterior (in front), are incorporated into the cast and protrude from the distal end. The anterior wire is bent forward and taped to the middle toe. The posterior wire is bent backward and taped to the posterior toe. These modifications adequately immobilise the foot, allowing the bone to heal. They are well accepted by the pigeon.

When the fracture occurs under the metal marking ring, trauma of the leg can cause swelling, with the ring interfering with circulation. The ring must be removed to prevent gangrene and necrosis, with resulting loss of the foot. If there is no swelling, strips of gypsona plaster are used and the ring is incorporated in the cast.
  Continued vigilance is required as the healing bone produces callus, which may cause circulatory disturbance one or two weeks following the accident. Unless the ring is removed, delayed gangrene of the foot follows .

On occasion both legs are broken. These cases are splinted or cast as described above, and confined to small cage. Alternatively the bird's legs are cast, or bound with bandage to prevent them swinging loosely and the pigeon confined to a hangmat, so placed that it has free access to food and water, without touching the ground. Pigeons accept this form of restraint very well. Two weeks of "bedrest" in a hangmat is adequate for fracture healing.

6.3. Tibial fractures.

Distal tibial fractures, near the hock joint, require immobilisation of the tibia, hock and proximal metatarsus. Gypsona plaster, applied in strips as described under fracture of the metatarsus, gives good results. It is essential that the hock is incorporated in the cast to prevent inward rotation of the leg when the pigeon lies down to rest.

Midline or proximal fractures of the tibia are immobilised with a splint made of adhesive tape (elastoplast) and a number of strips of wood, 3 cm.long. We prefabricate the splint, following which it is wrapped around the fractured part. A strip of tape, ±2.5 x 12 cm, is laid on a flat surface, adhesive side upwards. ± Eight wooden strips (match-size) are laid down on the central part of the tape, across the width and about 4mm. apart. The splint is now ready for application.

An assistant holds the pigeon while we fit the splint, which is done with the leg fully extended. For a left sided tibial fracture, the bird is held on its right side with its back toward the assistant. The assistant's left thumb pushes from in front, down on the bird's femur, forcing the leg towards the tail. This produces adequate extension of the leg and permits the operator to fit the splint. The splint is fitted in the midline of the tibia, above the hock. If the leg is defeathered to any extent, a thin layer of cotton wool is rolled onto the skin to serve as protection, over which the prepared slint is wrapped snugly. Wooden strips that are too long are trimmed and covered with adhesive tape. Additional tape is used to further secure the splint. Care must be taken that rotation of the foot does not occur during splinting. To prevent future rotation, the hock is incorporated into the splint with elastoplast.

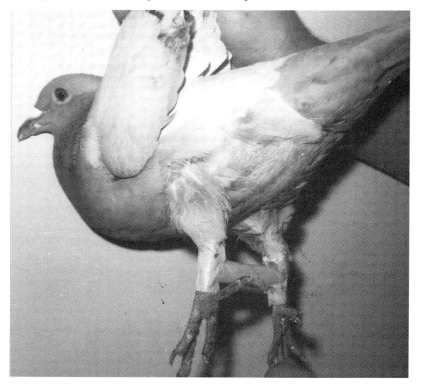

Bilateral fracture, the bird is double-splinted and will be slung in a hangmat. The bar between the legs prevents abnormal setting of the leg bones.

The wood-and-tape splint, the materials of which are always at hand, is light, cheap, quickly applied and very effective. A further advantage is its ease in removal – which can be a problem with a gypsona cast.

6.4. Femur fractures.

Femur fractures do not occur very often in pigeons and with the close proximity of the femur to the body, splinting is impractical. Other techniques must be employed.

If the fracture is simple, intramedullary pinning works well. However, this requires specialised equipment, anaesthesia of the patient, post-operative hospitalisation, is expensive and falls outside the needs of most fanciers. Because femur fractures heal easily – even if not immobilised, which can lead to healing in abnormal positions – temporary restraint, which is adequate to ensure recovery with full functional activity, is imposed. (Healing at abaxial angles takes place because when the pigeon lies down, resting his good leg, the injured leg is at an angle away from the body. The fractured bone grows on at this abnormal angle, usually at about 90° to the shaft of the femur.)

Sling rest

Restraint of uncontrolled movement of the fractured femur is achieved by restricting the pigeon to a sling or small hospital cage and anchoring the broken leg to the sound one. A short end of hard rubber or plastic tubing ± 3 cm. long, keeping the two legs parrallel, is fixed between the two metatarsals with adhesive tape. This allows the pigeon movement but prevents abaxial deviation of the fractured femur during the healing process.

Bilateral fractures of the metatarsal, tibial or femoral bones are best treated by splinting and hospitalisation in the sling. Food and water are provided and the birds are effectively prevented from using the broken legs. Pigeons accept the sling well and two weeks rest is long enough.

6.5. Wing fractures.

Serious fractures of the wing of a pigeon usually spell an end to its racing career. Although these fractures heal fairly well, some degree of muscle and joint stiffness nearly always results, leading to reduced racing ability. Simple fractures of the ulna can heal without serious consequences provided that the radius is intact.

Isolation and cage-rest for 20 days is sufficient treatment for ulnar fractures. We have seen pigeons win races following successful recovery from ulnar fracture.

Treatment of wing fractures consists of immobilising the wing onto the body in the normal resting position with strips of adhesive tape. Although the pigeons do not like it, they grudgingly endure adhesive bandage (Elastoplast) on their feathers for two to three weeks. A band of tape, 50 cm wide, is used. Taping begins high on the inside of the wing, runs down under the leading edge, up on the outside to go over the back and lift the wing, which usually droops slightly. Another strip of tape, about 3 cm. from the tip, fixes the primary flights together in the normal resting position to prevent their being dragged on the floor and becoming soiled and tattered.

Intramedullary pinning of bad wing fractures is essential to regain function but the end results are usually not good enough to allow the pigeon to further his racing career. Birds can be salvaged and retained for breeding purposes. The techniques for intramedullary pinning follow the standard procedures as applied in other species. We believe that invasion of joints by prosthetic materials, must be avoided, wherever possible. Detailed description of intramedullary pinning techniques, fall outside the scope of this book.

7. Caesarean section

7.1. Eggbinding

A pigeon, with a fully developed egg in the posterior oviduct, which it is struggling to lay, shows symptoms of respiratory distress and shock. If delivery, following the standard procedures, has failed, Caesarean section must be performed. The operation is relatively simple, safe and has a high rate of post-operative fertility.

The normal pre-operative routine is followed and a skin incision is made from the end of the sternum to 5 mm from the cloaca, taking care not to cut into the cloaca with subsequent soiling and infection of the wound. The deeper incision, through fat and peritoneum is made with care, ensuring that the oviduct is not prematurely entered. With the heavily-laden oviduct exposed, two stay sutures are placed on either side of the egg and the oviduct is incised between them. The egg is carefully removed but if too much difficulty is experienced with this procedure, the egg is punctured, sucked dry and the shell carefully removed. A continuous suture of 3/0 catgut repairs the oviduct. Peritoneum and muscle is sutured together and the third layer of sutures is placed in the skin.

Complete removal of the eggshell is essential, even if the egg breaks before or during surgery, as shell remnants cause a severe localised inflammation with subsequent fertility problems.

7.2. Yolk retention

Yolk retention is similar to eggbinding, insomuch as the yolk is not passed the full distance of the oviduct. Yolk retention is not discovered by the fancier for some time and the pigeon is usually brought for examination because it is no longer capable of laying. The inspissated yolk sits higher in the oviduct and is not as easily palpated. As the mass grows bigger, the bird shows more symptoms of not being well, with respiratory distress increasing. At this time serious (irreversible?) changes have already taken place in the oviduct lining, severely reducing the potential for future egg production.

The incision is made lateral to the breastbone in the left flank, from the last rib to 1 cm from the anus. This provides good access to the reproductive tract. The diseased oviduct is incised and the inspissated mass carefully shelled out.

Often the oviduct has been perforated, inspissated yolk has spilt into the abdomen and egg-yolk peritonitis is present. This drastically reduces the breeding potential. Antibiotics are instilled into the oviduct before closing the incision. Closure of the wound follows standard procedures.

8. Gastrotomy

Gastrotomy (incision into the muscular stomach) has to be performed on the rare occasions when pigeons have swallowed foreign objects like nails or bits of wire. These remain in the gizzard, which they penetrate causing peritonitis and abscesses. Having confirmed the diagnosis by radiographs (X-rays), an operation to remove the foreign object, and save the life of the bird, is performed. Lateral and ventro-dorsal radiographs are taken to demonstrate the position and direction of the offending object.

With the bird in dorsal recumbency an incision is made in the left abdominal wall, from behind the last rib almost to the anus. This provides good vision and access to the organs. The gizzard is identified. If the foreign object has penetrated through the posterior wall of the gizzard it is removed without further surgery. When opening the abdomen one must be aware that the offending nail is not visible, as the body has encapsulated it and an abscess has formed around it. In order to reach and extract the offending object, the abscess is incised, following which all abscessed material is removed.

If penetration has not occurred, the gizzard is fixed by means of two stay sutures and the wall of the organ is opened as widely as possible by blunt dissection, working in line with the direction of the muscle fibres. The horny internal layer is incised and the offending foreign object removed with a crocodile forceps or similar instrument. The gizzard muscle layer is closed with interrupted 3/0 catgut sutures. The abdominal muscle layers and skin are closed separately. Water is withheld for 12 hours and 24 hours later a small grain feed is offered. Recovery is uneventful.

9. Laparoscopy

Diagnostic laparoscopy is performed on a wide variety of bird species particularly for sexing purposes. In racing pigeons this is not necessary but laparoscopy may be performed for diagnostic purposes, where a number of diseases or organs may be involved. With a custom-designed endoscope the procedure is easy, rewarding and not stressful to the pigeon. The instrumentation however, is expensive and acquisition is not warranted for racing pigeon purposes. However a halogen-light-sourced auriscope may be used for the same purpose and is adequate in most instances.

The prime site for entry, is anterior to the vent bones, just behind the ribs. Left of the midline one enters the left abdominal airsac and from here the kidneys, adrenals, ureters, gonads and vasa deferentes may be seen. On the right side care must be taken to avoid injuring the small intestine. To view the liver, the optimal puncture site is midline, just distal to the sternum.

Having made a skin incision of 1.5 cm, the abdominal muscles are parted by blunt dissection and the peritoneum is incised. The speculum of the auriscope is introduced and the required examinations performed. Upon completion the skin is sutured with or one two interrupted sutures.

8. Abdominal hernia

Abdominal hernia usually occurs in old and overweight breeding hens. There is some belief that abdominal hernia interferes with egglaying but an obese pigeon will have difficulty in laying – whether or not a hernia is present. Provided the herniation is not yet massive, with large-scale muscle tissue destruction, correction is effective. Prevention depends mainly on dietary control and management.

Damage to muscle fibres begins at a young age, but is insignificant and passes undetected. The straining effects of egg-laying are cumulative and once the process is begun, is difficult to stop, because the original causes are usually entrapped within the management. With more muscle fibres losing their anatomical structure and separating from each other, muscle tears gradually become larger. Abdominal hernias predominantly occur in old hens because of the cumulative damage of pressure, brought about by many laying periods. The harmful side-effects of laying are markedly increased if the hen is overweight, unfit and fed a deficient diet.

Operative Procedure

The skin is incised over the herniated area (which occurs on or adjacent to the midline) and the herniated material, usually fat, is gently returned to the abdomen or resected. The hernia ring is cleared of fat and the edges freshened and sutured together (3/0 catgut). The skin incision is sutured with 3/0 nylon or similar material.

When multiple hernias occur together, one's chances of successful intervention are decreased.

• DRUGS AND MEDICATION •

Chapter 16

Administration and dosing

A great deal of the information in this section is scattered about elsewhere in the book but has been summarised and combined with other relevant details in this chapter.

Administration of medicines.

When individual pigeons are presented for treatment, a choice must be made between oral or parenteral administration.

Injectable administration.

Injections are generally safe. The intramuscular route into the breast muscles is used for nonracing pigeons whereas the subcutaneous route is preferred for racers.

The back of the neck is the preferred site for subcutaneous injection, midway between the head and 'shoulders'. A right-handed injector works as follows. Holding the bird in the customary position with his right hand, an assistant grasps the head with his left, pulling it forward towards him and straightening the neck. The injector lifts a few feathers at the back of the neck, finds a visible patch of bare skin and injects in a forward direction towards the head. The skin is penetrated for no more that 3 to 5 mm. Entry into the crop, cervical airsac and other sensitive areas must be avoided.

Intramuscular injection is done with the pigeon held horizontally on its back. The feathers covering the pectoral muscles are brushed aside and the needle is inserted forward and downward for 10 to 15 mm. A damaged vein results in severe bleeding, with discolouration of the tissues for three weeks and longer.

Oral administration

Individual oral treatment is accomplished by dosing with capsules, tablets or liquid. It is easier if an assistant holds the bird. The left hand of the doser holds the head and opens the beak, while the right doses the medicine. It is possible to do this singlehandedly by resting the bird on a table, imprisoning it against one's body and simultaneously opening the beak with the thumb and forefinger of the holding hand. The free hand is used to administer the medicine.

Oral medication has the disadvantage that the time period till availability of the medicine is variable and depends on the amount of food in the crop. In liquid medicines the active ingredient is available directly, once past the gizzard. A few medicines are absorbed from the crop. Pills and capsules release their ingredients in the crop, or, if not dissolved or digested, in the gizzard. In fasting birds a pill (capsule), passes almost immediately to the gizzard, whereas a full crop retards the passage from the crop.

Most tablets and pills are designed for mammals with a specific digestion time, allowing release of the active substance in a particular area of the digestive system. Release of medicine in the crop, may result in vomiting and loss of medicine. Sugar-coated tablets pass the crop and release their content in the gizzard. Individual treatment requires extra time and effort.

Mass dosing of pigeons is best done by medicating the drinking water. Occasionally the feed is sprinkled with vitamin powders, Brewer's Yeast powder, flowers of sulphur or one of the nitrofurans. Where the safety margin is narrow, this method is not recommended because unequal distribution through the feed may result in unequal uptake, causing intoxication.

Large-scale dosing via the water bowl, which is preferably made of glass or some similar inert, non-scratch material, is accepted practice. The birds will readily take medicated water, even if it is a strange colour, salty or very bitter to human taste. Birds detest sour-tasting water. If doctoring leaves the water with a strong smell, the pigeons will approach nervously at first but once the boldest has drunk, the rest will follow.

The amount of water consumed by pigeons in a specific day is variable and depends on the climatic conditions, activity of the birds and stage of rearing and complicates this method.

During an average sunny winter day, racing pigeons in training will drink approximately 50 ml. water. On hot days this amount will increase to 100 ml, or more. Birds with large babies in the nest will take up 100 ml. and even double this amount on hot days. On cold, rainy days, water consumption may drop to 20 or 25 ml. per day.

Birds on eggs drink less than pigeons rearing large youngsters. It is advisable, therefore, that the breeding cycles of all birds coincide to some extent.

The tremendous variation in water consumption must be brought into reckoning when medications are given via the water trough. Several methods are used to ensure correct dosages.

The total amount of medicine, calculated for one day, is added to the total amount of water, estimated to be consumed on that day and given to the birds.

The total amount of medicine, calculated for one day, is added to less water than the birds will require on that day and given to the birds. Unmedicated water is provided once the medicated water has been drunk. Medicated water is preferably given following meals.

A less accurate method, but easier to apply, is used in practice. The total amount of water drunk per day is estimated (50 ml per pigeon) and the calculated amount of medicine added to it. (This amount of water may be below average for our local conditions, particularly in summer.) Usually this concentration is then given for the period. Unmedicated water may be given if the conditions change drastically.

Accuracy of dosage is important with some medicines eg. dimetridazole (Emtryl), an overdosage of which causes marked nervous symptoms, and less so with others eg. metronidazole (Flagyl), which has a wide safety margin and in which overdosage is rarely seen. Antibiotic over- or underdosage is usually not so critical, provided that the incorrect dosage is not continued for longer than one or two days, as long-term treatment at incorrect levels cause severe problems.

Note:

1. We do not weigh every individual pigeon but use an average

body mass of 500 g. per bird, to calculate the various dosages. Variations from this figure may be marked but water intake is usually relative to body mass. For cases treated individually, the necessary adjustments must be made.

2. In all cases antibacterials are administered for a minimum of three days but administration may be prolonged, up to six weeks, in some instances.

3. For prolonged treatment a lower dose is usually recommended.

4. Dosages may vary from those in other publications. Varying dosages result from different experiences or different opinions regarding preventative treatment. Our philosophy regarding dosages may be controversial:

4.1. For the obviously sick bird: The dose as given, applies.

4.2. For the subclinically sick bird (carrier): To eradicate the disease the FULL dose is recommended.

4.3. For the unexposed birds: The birds cannot be kept healthy in the future by prophylactic treatment in the present. (No treatment advised).

4.4. For the exposed birds; Exposed healthy stock are only protected by treatment while they are being treated. Once the protection of treatment has ceased, (usually after 12-24 hours) the birds again become fully susceptible. They are, however, protected by treatment if the treatment cures the subclinical birds (carriers), and they are no longer exposed!

5. Antibiotics used as growth stimulants for chickens, pigs, etc. are fed at a low dosage for protracted periods. Their use here does not apply and does not warrant discussion.

6. The absolute correctness of a dose is not essential. If it were, no medicines could be administered via the drinking water, because of the variable consumption.

Dosages are readily measured in teaspoons, i.e. measuring (medical) teapoons with a slight rounding of the medicinial powder content, neither heaped nor scraped off flat. As a general rule we assume that such a teapoon holds 4g (gram) powder. (Some powders are heavier and others lighter but the variation is not statistically significant). Where absolutely correct measures are essential, it is recommended that a scale is used or that the product is administered individually, orally or by injection.

Reasons for failure of a given medicine.

1. Probably the most common reason for treatment failure, is underdosage, which results from;
    a) inadequate dosage
    b) inadequate dosage interval
    c) inadequate duration of treatment
    d) any combination of all three above.

2. Varying concentrations of the given medicine in specific organs or systems. This especially true for the poorly absorbed drugs and some antibiotics. For example, tylosin concentration is higher in lung, liver and kidneys, than in plasma. A plasma concentration figure would therefore give a distorted picture.

3. Over-reliance on medications. Medicine often has to be given in conjunction with other procedures or a change in management.

Precautions to bear in mind.

One must always attempt to prevent the appearance of resistant organisms by;
    a) using suitable dosage regimens
    b) beginning treatment early
    c) continuing treatment long enough
    d) avoiding the use of antibiotics for minor illnesses (racing results!)
    e) monititoring progress via regular laboratory testing (impractical).

Chapter 17

Antibiotics and racing

Fallacies about medicines, particularly about antibiotics, abound amongst fanciers. Although it is true that some antibiotics tend to be more concentrated in certain areas of the body, their effect is on germs and not on organs. An antibiotic therefore must not be seen as good for a particular organ but rather as active against the germs that commonly occur in such an organ.

Whatever is said about antibiotics, applies equally well to the antibacterials – eg. sulphonamides. They are similar, the main difference being that antibiotics were originally produced by micro-organisms (some are now manufactured synthetically) and antibacterials are purely synthetic.

More and more use is made of antibiotics in pigeon racing. Occasionally the use of the drugs is justified, as when explicit disease is present, but more and more frequently they are given because of the mistaken belief that antibiotics are some kind of stimulant, making the birds perform above their natural physical capabilities. This is a fallacy, as there are no drugs (steroid hormones included), that will enable healthy in-form pigeons to win races that they could not otherwise win.

Antibiotics can, if given correctly, assist the bird to achieve maximum health and by this means improve performances. There are many disease conditions that negatively affect pigeon super health. Being strong and resilient creatures, (selection through decades of racing has helped immensely), the revealing signs of ill-health are hidden beneath a cloak of apparent health and only scientific tests can reveal the truth. The trained eye of an experienced fancier detects that something is preventing 'form', but often he does not know just what it is.

When these birds are given the correct medicine a resulting

burst of good health follows, during which time races may be won. This is not owing to the medicine but to the sudden acquisition of top condition. If repeated the next week, the race results are often disappointing.

All drugs have side-effects and when healthy pigeons are dosed with antibiotics they are handicapped. No medicine is totally harmless to the host. Although the concentrated effect is aimed against the invading germ, some side-effects are experienced by the host. How can it possibly improve racing potential in a healthy specimen?

Side-effects include the following:

1. Reactions may occur in specific systems of the body. The gastro-intestinal tract, particularly the liver and intestine, urogenital tract, haemopoetic (blood-forming) and nervous systems may experience idiosyncratic episodes from drug use. Included amongst these are manifestations of hypersensitivity reactions.

2. Oral administration causes suppression of normal bacterial flora of the intestine, and can lead to fungal overgrowth if given over extended periods.

3. Vitamin B12 synthesis is inhibited in mammals and may lead to vitamin deficiency. Many rodents and most herbivores rely on bacterial fermentation for normal digestion. Oral antibiotics can be fatal to these species. The normal intestinal bacterial population of pigeons has not been adequately studied and some controversy exists as to whether oral antibiotics are detrimental to these birds.

4. Constant use of antibiotics, particularly if underdosed, can promote the development of bacterial resistance. This can be chromosomal resistance, which is transmissible to suceeding generations or plasmid determined resistance, which can be transmitted to other, non-related bacteria.

In practice it means that when a fancier administers antibiotics to his birds to promote their racing ability, he may excite the formation of plasmid resistance in non-pathogenic bacteria. These are capable of transmitting their acquired resistance to pathogenic bacteria and subsequent antibiotic administration to combat the pathogenic organisms, will be ineffective. I believe that this has already occurred in some germs, that have developed plasmid resistance to the tetracyclines.

In pigeons, little work has been done on the absorption and excretion of antibiotics, with minimal work published on the level and duration of adequate blood-levels (MIC) following administration.

'Interesting' practices, (in other words, fanciers are warned not to fall into the same trap), followed with antibiotics, include; .

1. Dosages are unknown or if known, are executed inaccurately and when failures occur the drugs, and not the dosages are blamed. Dosages applicable to poultry or mammals cannot always be employed for pigeons. They are a different species with different reactions and though satisfactory results are sometimes obtained, on other occasions they are not.

2. Following treatment, most fanciers assume that the disease treated for, is eradicated and post-treatment testing is rarely done. If no response to treatment is seen, it is assumed that the disease was misdiagnosed. Rarely is the dosage or the method of administration questioned. Occasionally the medicine itself is declared ineffective.

3. Efficacy of treatment is usually measured against positions obtained in the first subsequent race. At the least, substantial improvement is desired. Little time is allowed for the birds to recover from the stress of the disease or the side-effects of drug treatment.

Recent work, investigating bloodlevels following different administration routes and dosages, discovered unknown facts but raises new questions. Eg.: chloramphenicol after an oral dose of 200 mg per kg. was found not to give 'therapeutic' bloodlevels. If chloramphenicol given by oral suspension at 200 mg/kg provides significant clinical improvement of the disease syndrome what do 'therapeutic' bloodlevels mean? Is the therapeutic blood level of chloramphenicol in pigeons different to that of mammals? If so, a whole new field of research is opened, especially if the premise applies also to other antibiotics.

Other problems exist for the pigeon fancier attempting to use antibiotics correctly. Because the market for antibiotics used in pigeons is relatively small, few drug companies market medicines exclusively for use in pigeons. With a few exceptions the drugs used by fanciers are spin-offs from the poultry or other animal industries. Dosages are not given for pigeons, nor is mention made of disease problems in pigeons. Few scientists have a working knowledge of the medicines as administered to pigeons and though the situation is slowly improving, vast areas are still to be researched. Fanciers are limited, for a working knowledge of dosages, to friends the few specialist veterinarians with previous dosage experience, petshops, salesmen, pharmacies, trial and error or blind guesswork.

Besides the trade names of antibiotics, sulphonamides, nitrofurans and other drugs mentioned in this book, there are other preparations on the market, of which a quick study will reveal that most of them have the same active ingredient(s). These countless mixtures and concoctions are available under a wide variety of trade names. Many of these are imported by petshops and dealers. To protect his pigeons and obtain effective treatment, the fancier is obligated to read and recognise (memorise) the ingredients. Though usually safe, there is little benefit in trying the same drug under a different trade name if it was ineffective the first time.

For example if Terramycin, an antibiotic, active ingredient (generic name) oxytetracycline, fails to achieve the desired effect, Contromycin, also containing oxytetracycline, cannot improve on Terramycin.

Similarly 5-Amino-nitrothiazole (generic name) is sold under the trade names Harkanka, Enheptine, Entramin, Tricoxine and Tricoxitab. If one fails to effect treatment, the other four are unlikely to do any better. To try them would be a waste of time, money and effort.

Chapter 18

Antimicrobials

1. The antibiotics

An attempt is made, for each drug, to give the correct dosage rate (to establish the Required blood-level or MIC = Minimum Inhibitary Concentration). The total dosage per day is given, and may be administered in two or three divided doses. The abbreviations in the dosage suggestions refer to the following methods of application: (i.m.) refers to intramuscular injection; (p.o.) refers to being given orally and (s/c) refers to subcutaneous injection.

Included here are those products and trade names known at the time of writing. Changes in pharmaceutical companies' marketing and sales strategies will mean that, inevitably, some products are not longer available and some new ones introduced. Others will be marketed by different companies or under different names. In some countries some of the following drugs may not be available or may not be available for specific use in pigeons. However it is important that a broad overview of the antimicrobial products used on pigeons be given as what is unavailable in one country may be freely sold in another. If you are uncertain about which drugs are available, or which are available under a different trade name, then consult a veterinarian who has an interest in avian or pigeon disease.

AMOXYCILLIN

Dosage Rate; 100-150 mg/kg (i.m.); 100-150 mg/kg (p.o.)

Generic name	Trade name	Present	Marketing Co	Dosage
Amoxycillin	Clamoxyl	inject	SmithKl.Beecham	50mg/bird
	Clamoxyl PP	SP	SmithKl.Beecham	1g/litre

In combination with

Tylosin	Longstim	SP	Medpet	5g/litre

Notes – Effective against Salmonella.
   – Twice as rapidly excreted by pigeons as by mammals.
   – Good availability after intramuscular injection.
   – Cross resistance between ampicillin and amoxycillin.

AMPICILLIN

Dosage Rate; 100-150 mg/kg (i.m.); 100-150 mg/kg (p.o.)

Generic name	Trade name	Present	Marketing Co	Dosage
Ampicillin	Ampill-Vet 100	inject	Kruger-Med	1ml/10kg

Notes – Effective against Salmonella.
   – Twice as rapidly excreted by pigeons as by mammals.
   – Good availability after intramuscular injection.
   – Cross resistance between ampicillin and amoxycillin.
   – Erratic absorption following oral administration – affected
     by food in the gut.

CHLORAMPHENICOL

Dosage Rate; 40-80 mg/kg (i.m.); 1g/litre (p.o.)

Chloramphenicol has been used extensively against paratyphoid although some studies have shown it to be of limited value against the disease.
   Published work (AVMA Journal, 1982) has shown that an intramuscular injection at 100 mg per kg provided therapeutic blood levels for less than three hours. The same study revealed that therapeutic concentrations were not achieved following the highest oral dose given i.e. 200 mg per kg given once daily. In contrast we experienced clinical response following oral administration of the drug. Plasmid related transmissable resistance to chloramphenicol has been seen.

Generic name	Trade name	Present	Marketing Co	Dosage
Chloramphenicol	Chl'phenicol10%	inject	Panvet	0.5ml/kg s/c
Chloramphenicol	Chloramphenicol SP	SP	CE Indust.	2-4g/litre

In combination with

Oxytetracycline	Controbac	inject	Truka-Panvet	0.5ml/kg

Oxytetracycline + Prednisolone	Controbac-Vet	inject	Panvet	0.5ml/kg
Na arsanilate + vitamins	Chloramphenicol +	SP	Chevita	1pkt/lit

ERYTHROMYCIN

Dosage Rate; 40-50 mg/kg (i.m.)

Used occasionally in the treatment of throat infections. Narrow-spectrum, bacteriostatic – not active against mycoplasma in vitro. Used extensively in combination with other drugs eg. Mycosan-T (Chevita) and Tylo-Tad Plus (Phenix). High levels of concentration occur in the lungs.

Generic name	Trade name	Present	Marketing Co	Dosage
Erythromycin In combination with Tylosin + Furaltadone+vits	Tylo-Tad Plus	SP	Phenix	2g/litre
Arsanilic acid+ vits	Mycosan-T	SP	Chevita	1pkt/1-2litres

Arsanilic acid is a narrow-spectrum antibiotic and is occasionally used as a growth stimulant

GENTOMYCIN

Dosage Rate; 3-7 mg/kg (i.m.)

Very potent. Overdosage can cause renal toxicity.

LINCOMYCIN

Dosage Rate; 100 mg/kg (i.m.).

Lincomycin is safe for use in pigeons. It is a narrow-spectrum antibiotic with maximal activity against Gram-positive organisms. Used extensively for control of respiratory infections in pigeons, particularly active against mycoplasmas but not active against Chlamydia psittaci.

Generic name	Trade name	Present	Marketing co	Dosage
Lincomycin HCl	Lincocin CT 200	Inject	Upjohn	1ml/kg s/c

In combination with

Spectinomycin	Lincospectin 12,5%	SP	Upjohn	4-5g/litre

NEOMYCIN

Dosage Rate; 100 mg/kg. (p.o.)

Neomycin is used especially in combinations with other antibiotics and because it is poorly absorbed from the intestine its use in pigeons is restricted to intestinal conditions. Potentially toxic the drug may cause disturbances of the auditory and vestibular organs when used in injectable form.

Generic name	Trade name	Present	Marketing Co	Dosage
Neomycin	Neophen	SP	Phenix	1g/2litre

In combination with;

Oxytetracycline	Neo-terramycin	SP	Pfizer	2.5g/litre
Oxytetracycline	Neo-troxine	SP	Rhone-Poulenc	2g/litre

PENICILLIN

The first antibiotic discovered. Still used extensively in veterinary and human medicine. Gram-negative organisms have a natural resistance. Various gram-positive organisms have developed resistance in different forms and have neccesitated the development of bio-synthetic and semi-synthetic penicillins. Usually combined with streptomycin to broaden their spectrum.

   Use of natural penicillin (acid labile) is limited in pigeons to the injectable forms. No penetration of the CSF and excreted virtually unchanged in the urine.

Dosage Rate; +20 000 iu/kg (s.c.) (1 iu=0.6 mcg)

Generic name	Trade name	Present	Marketing Co	Dosage
Injectable				
Benzylpenicillin	Peni 30M	Inject	Phenix	1ml/30kg
	Depocillin	Inject	Intervet	0.1ml/kg
Penicillin G	Proc. Penicillin G	Inject	Milborrow	0.1ml/kg

in combination with;

Streptomycin	Streptopen	Inject	Milborrow	0.1ml/kg

QUINOLONE CARBOLIC ACID DERIVATIVES

A new group of antibiotics that is claimed to be effective against mycoplasma spp. in chickens, E. coli and salmonella. Cross-resistance is found within the quinolone group. Plasmid transmissible resistance has not been seen.

Generic Name	Trade Name	Present	Marketing Co	Dosage
Enrofloxacin	Baytril	liquid	Bayer	1-2ml/2l
Danofloxacin	Advocin	SP	Pfizer	1g/1-2l

SPECTINOMYCIN

Dosage Rate; 20mg/kg (p.o.); 5-10 mg/kg (i.m.)

Poorly absorbed (7%) from the gastro-intestinal tract. Effective against several mycoplasma spp. Used as soluble powder (Lincospectin) in combination with Lincomycin at dosage rate 1-2g/litre water.

Generic name	Trade name	Present	Marketing Co	Dosage
Spectinomycin	Salmosan-t	inject	Chevita	0.5ml/pgn

SPIRAMYCIN

Spiramycin enjoys popularity in Europe as part of various mixtures for the treatment of upper respiratory diseases. Sold under the trade name, Suanovil, it has a narrow-spectrum of activity.

STREPTOMYCIN

Dosage Rate; 30-75 mg/kg (s/c)

Streptomycin is poorly absorbed from the gut and its use orally in infections other than enteritis, is questionable. In injectable form it has some benefit on respiratory infections. It has a stressful effect on pigeons causing them to lose consciousness at overdose. It is nephrotoxic and ototoxic.

Historically used in pigeons in injection form at dosage rate

200mg/kg (20 x overdose). Birds suffered vasomotor collapse but a good response was reported upon recovery from collapse (measured in subsequent racing success). Whether improvement was owing to elimination of the mycoplasmas or from the shock reaction is unknown.

Generic Name	Trade Name	Present	Marketing Co	Dosage
Dihydrostrep-	Distrep	inject	Milborrow	25mg/kg
tomycin	DHS 250	inject	Phenix	25mg/kg

in combination with;

Penicillin	Pendistrep 20/20	inject	Phenix	0.25ml/kg

Streptomycin in injectable form is particularly useful in combination with penicillin, though the treatment intervals for the two drugs is different and poses a problem. The calculated dosage of streptomycin and twice the calculated dosage for the penicillin is given.

Pendistrep 2ml (streptomycin and penicillin) is made up to 10 ml with water. 0.5ml of the diluted solution is injected subcutaneously at the back of the neck, twice daily. Good results have been obtained in valuable birds with non-specific infections, particularly when the bird is too ill to drink medicated water.

TETRACYCLINES

Dosage Rate; 90 mg/kg (p.o.)

The tetracyclines have been extensively used in pigeon medicine. The group includes tetracycline, oxy-, roli- and chlortetracycline, and doxycycline. For many years the tetracyclines were the only products in use against Chlamydia (Ornithosis) and mycoplasmas, and Terramycin (oxytetracycline) was widely used by pigeon fanciers, sometimes incorrectly as stimulant sometimes on a one-day-per-week basis. As a result, resistance has built up to the drug and Terramycin has lost much of its value.

Some of the more commonly available preparations for pigeon use are :

Generic name	Trade name	Present	Marketing Co	Dosage
Oxytetracycline	Engemycine 10 %	inject	Intervet SA	1ml/kg
	Terramycin	inject	Pfizer	2ml/kg
	Oxycycline	inject	Truka-Panvet	1ml/kg
	Miltet	inject	Milborrow	2ml/kg

	Contromycin	SP	Truka-Panvet	5g/2l
	Liquamycin AF	SP	Pfizer	5g/2l
	Oxytracycline SP	SP	Anchorpharm	5g/2l
	Ph'x Oxyphen 20%	SP	Phenix	1g/2l
Chlortetracycline	Chlortetracyclin+	SP	Chevita	1pkt/1-2l
Tetracycline	Polyotic	SP	Kruger-Med	5g/2l
Doxycycline	Doxymycin QA	inject	Milborrow	0.1ml/kg
	Mildox	inject	Milborrow	0.1ml/kg
	Dovabiotic	tablets	Dova	1tab/pgn
Tetracycline in combination with;				
Oleandomycine	Sigmamycine	SP	Pfizer	8g/5l
Oxytetracycline in combination with;				
vitamins	Liquamycin + vits	SP	Pfizer	5g/2l
	Terravit + vits	SP	Pfizer	5g/2l
	Phenix Oxyvit	SP	Phenix	5g/2l
Furazolidone	Kemtrox WD	SP	Rhone-Poulenc	2-4g/l
Furazolidone, Furaltadone+vits	Oxyvital	SP	Phenix	2-4g/l
Neomycin	Neo-Terramycin	SP	Pfizer	2g/l
	Neo-Troxine	SP	Rhone-Poulenc	2g/l
Oleandomycin	Sigmamycin	SP	Pfizer	1-2g/l
Doxycycline in combination with;				
vitamins	Doxybiotic	SP	Medpet	5g/l

Notes 1. The effective clinical injectable dose of oxytetracycline for pigeons exceeds the mammalian dose and has no side-effects.

2. Calcium has an affinity for the tetracyclines and shell-grit needs to be withdrawn when the drug is given orally. Failure to do so results in the drug being bound to the

calcium, preventing its uptake into the system.

3. Doxycycline has better bloodlevels than the tetracyclines because of active reabsorption takes place from the gut following excretion by the liver. Doxycycline uptake is not affected by the presence of calcium.

4. Doxycycline has a halflife of 20 hours and needs only to be given once in 24 hours. Is antibiotic of choice for treating ornithosis.

5. Special care is taken with oxytetracycline as the injection is irritant and necrotising to the tissues. Subcutaneous injections are safer than intramuscular.

5. Tetracyclines are effective against chlamydia (Ornithosis) and mycoplasmas.

TIAMULIN

Dosage Rate; 25 mg/kg (p.o.)

Active against mycoplasmas but resistance develops in these organisms. Causes severe feather abnormalties when given at excessive dosages during the moulting season. Used by fanciers – water soluble form – in the drinking water. Causes acute mortalities at four times the recommended dosage rate.

Dosage Rate; 12-15 mg/kg (p.o.)

Generic name	Trade name	Present	Marketing Co	Dosage
Tiamulin	Tiamutin 45 %	SP	Milborrow	1-2g/litre
	Tiamutin	soln	Leo labs	2ml/litre

TYLOSIN

Dosage Rate; 50 mg/kg (p.o.)

Tylosin has been inherited from the poultry industry where it is particularly succesful against the mycoplasmas. The oral forms of the have drug has been used by racing pigeon fanciers to treat pigeons for conditions of the respiratory tract, particularly ornithosis and mixed infections.
  Not very soluble. Mix with warm water before adding to rest of

drinking water.

Generic name	Trade name	Present	Marketing Co	Dosage
Tylosin	Tylan Soluble	SP	Elanco	1g/litre
	Tylosin Tart PP	SP	Phenix	1g/litre

In combination with;
Erythromycin +

Furaltadone+vits	Tylo-tad	SP	Phenix	2.5g/litre
Chlortetracycline	Tylosin Plus	SP	Chevita	1pkt/1-2lit

2. The Nitrofurans

The nitrofurans are historically well-known to most older fanciers through trade names such as Bifuran and Furasol and many pigeons have been nursed to health and greater glory by the judicious use of these drugs. The nitrofurans are particularly effective against the gut-active bacteria and are used mainly against salmonellosis (in combination with antibiotics) and secondary infections. Nervous symptoms arise from overdosage with nitrofurans, especially when given in conjunction with dimetridazole (Emtryl – used against hexamitiasis). Young birds are susceptible to excessive intake of the combination.

The nitrofurans are not active against coccidiosis.

Dosage Rate; (furaltadone) 15-20 mg/kg (p.o.); (furazolidone) 15-20 mg/kg (p.o.)

Generic name	Trade name	Present	Marketing Co	Dosage
Furaltadone	Furaltadone 28.5 %	SP	Phenix	1g/litre
	Furaltadone 13,2 %	SP	Anchorpharm	2g/litre
	Furasol 20%	SP	Sm.Kl. Beecham	2-4g/litre
Furazolidone	Kemzol FP	SP	Phenix	2-4g/litre
	Neftin	tablet	Smith Kline	.12 tab bd
	Coryzium	capsule	Harkers	1caps/bird
	Furazolidon+	SP	Chevita	1pkt/2litres

In combination with;

Oxytetracycline	Kemtrox WD	SP	Maybaker	2-4g/litre

Oxytetracycline

+ vitamins	Oxyvital	SP	Phenix	2.5g/litre

| Tylosin +, Erythromycin +vits | Tylo-Tad Plus | SP | Phenix | 2.5g/litre |
| Arsanilic acid+ vits+minerals | Furazolidon+ | SP | Chevita | 1pkt/2litres |

3. The sulphonamides

Simple Sulphonamides

The sulphonamides are widely used as antimicrobials and are particularly valuable for treating and controlling coccidiosis. In pigeons it is currently recommended that treatment for coccidiosis must be continued for 7 to 10 days. (Poultry are treated on a 3 – 2 – 3 schedule.) Reinfection of the flock is prevented by sanitising the loft with a chlorine product or by singe-cleansing with a flame. Historically the sulphonamides were used against paratyphoid with varying success.

- Bacterial resistance readily develops and is effective against ALL the sulphonamides.

- The simple sulphonamides can cause depigmentation of the growing feathers when given to young birds 10 to 12 days old.

- Sulphonamides can cause rough- and thin-shelled eggs.

- Some sulphonamides are poorly absorbed and have their greatest activity in the gastro-intestinal tract. For example Sulphaquinoxaline (Embazin) is a gut-active sulphonamide used widely for coccidiosis. Minimal absorption from the intestine. Sulphathiazole (Avisol) is widely used for respiratory infections but its potency is doubtful as the sulpha is poorly absorbed from the gut. Also useful for coccidiosis.

Generic name	Trade name	Present	Marketing Co	Dosage
Sulphadimidine	S'mezathine 16%	liquid	Hoechst	15ml/litre
Sulphadimidine	Sulfazine 16%	liquid	Milborrow	15ml/litre
Sulphadimidine	Dovasulf	liquid	Dova	20ml/litre
Sulphaquinoxaline	Embazin	liquid	Rhone-Poulenc	4ml/litre
	Quinox	soln	Microbiologicals	4ml/litre

Sulphathiazole	Avisol	liquid	Rhone-Poulenc	15ml/litre
S'chloropyrazine	ESB3	SP	Aesculap	1g/litre
	ESB3	SP	Ciba-Geigy	1g/litre

Generic name	Trade name	Present	Marketing Co	Dosage
In combination; Sulphamerazine+ Sulphamezathine+ S'thiazole+vits	Triple Sulfa	SP	Solvay	1g/2litres
Sulphathiazole+ Sulphadiazine+ Sulphamerazine	Trimeto Tad	SP	Phenix	5g/litre
Sulphadimidine+ Amprolium+vits	Sulphamezathin+	SP	Chevita	1pkt/ 2litres

Potentiated sulphonamides

Potentiated sulphonamides are sulphonamides combined with other drugs to produce a synergistic effect, in which the antimicrobial activity of the combination is greater than that of the two separately. Trimethoprim in particular, is used to combine with various sulphonamides.

The combinations are well-established for veterinary use but are only occasionally used for the treatment of pigeon disorders and then mainly when individual birds are treated.

Potentiated sulphonamides have a tendency to cause depigmentation of young growing feathers

Dosage Rate; (Tribissen) 1mg/kg (i.m.)

Generic name	Trade name	Present	Marketing Co	Dosage
with Trimethoprim				
S'methoxypyridazine	Coli-mix +	SP	Anchorpharm	1g/4litres
S'chlorpyridazine	Cosumix plus	SP	Ciba-Geigy	1g/litre
S'monomethoxine	Daimeton WS+	SP	Rhone-Poulenc	10g/litre
S'chlorpyridazine	Coli-Rid Oral	SP	Solvay	1ml/litre
S'quinoxaline	Whitsyn S	liquid	Beecham	1.5ml/litre

4. The protozoicides

Trichomoniasis, coccidiosis and pseudomalaria occur frequently
and modern pigeon racing hinges on the successful use of protozoi-
cides. The available drugs are safe, easy to administer, cheap and
effective.

4.1 Coccidiostats

Coccidiosis is arguably the most devastating of the pigeon
diseases, in spite of being poorly understood and intensive
research is needed before it can be treated with confidence. From
work in the poultry industry we know that all sulphonamides are
effective in the control of coccidiosis and they are widely used in
pigeon treatment schedules.

For a summary of the sulphonamides popularly used, the reader
must refer to the tables on sulphonamides in this chapter.
Sulphamezathine 16%, Sulfazine, Salsbury Triple Sulpha,
Embazin, ESB3 and Chevita's Sulphamezathin are the more
commonly-used formulations. For the treatment of coccidiosis one
sulpha drug does not have any superiority over another.

New coccidiostats are continually being developed and the
following are now also widely used:

Generic name	Trade name	Present	Marketing Co	Dosage
Toltrazuril	Baycox	liquid	Bayer AH	1ml/litre
Clazuril	Appertex	tablet	Janssen	1 tablet per pigeon
Amprol 20%	Amprolium	SP	Logos Agvet	1-2g/litre

4.2 Flagellicides

The only flagellate protozoa of pathologic significance are
Trichomonas and Hexamita. Clinical control by various flagellicides is effective but carrier states are not always eliminated.

Generic name	Trade name	Present	Marketing Co	Dosage
Dimetridazole	Emtryl SP	SP	Rhone-Poulenc	a) 5g/8litres b) 4g/2litres
	Gabbrocol	SP	Chevita	1pkt/litres
	Dovatric	liquid	Dova	5ml/litres
	Dovatric	tablets	Dova	1 tablet pigeon repeat in 4 d

	Trykil	SP	Norvet	1pkt/4litres
Metronidazole	Flagyl	tablet	Rhone-Poulenc	quarter tablet per pigeon
	Flagyl	liquid	Rhone-Poulenc	20ml/litre
	Meditrich	tablet	Medpet	1 tablet per pigeon
	Adco-metronidazole	tablet	Adco Pharm	half tablet per pigeon
Carnidazole	Spartrix	tablet	Janssen	1 tablet per pigeon
	Spartrix	tablet	Harkers	1 tablet per pigeon
Ronidazole	Tricho Plus	SP	Oropharma	1 teaspoon per 2 litres
	Sprint-geel	SP	Profarma	1pkt/2.5litres
Ridzol-S	SP		MSD-AGVET	1g/1-2l
Aminonitro-thiazole	Aminotrol	tablet		1 tablet per pigeon
	Harkanka	capsule	Harkers	1 capsule per pigeon
	Tricoxine	capsule	Fabry	1 capsule per pigeon
	Tricoxitab	tablet	Fabry	1 tablet per pigeon

Notes:

1. Emtryl (dimetridazole): two dosages are used against trichomonas.
   a). Preseason – with the birds resting – give for 7 days.
   b). In racing season – give for three days only.

2. Metronidazole (Emtryl) used in combination with a nitrofuran against hexamitiasis.

Dose: Emtryl, 5 g per 8 litres; Furazolidone, 2 g per litre.

Nervous symptoms are sometimes a side effect of the combination treatment.

2. Metronidazole (Emtryl) is toxic at overdose. Signs of toxicity include nervous symptoms, such as head tilt, blindness, torticollis, inability to fly as usual and loss of balance. Overdosage occurs with excessive water intake eg. pigeons feeding babies in the nest, particularly on hot days or with birds suffering from paramyxovirosis.

Treatment: Exchange medicated water for fresh water and do not disturb. Recovery follows.

3. Amino-nitrothiazole allows the development of more pathogenic strains by inhibiting less virulent strains, which control numbers of pathogenic strain. (Competition for food and space?).

4. Research is needed to examine the effect of herpes virus infection on the persistence of trichomonas ingection following treatment. We have repeatedly treated the same pigeons against trichomonas with various standard remedies and have found resistent infection, which disappeared co-incident with receding signs of herpes infection.

4.3 Others

Trade name	Generic name	Present	Marketing Co.	Dosage
Antemal	Primequine	liquid	Bluebird 2ml/litre	10 days

Chapter 19

Parasiticides

1. Anthelmintics

All the anthelmintics used in pigeons were developed primarily for use in other species as pigeons were considered too insignificant a group to warrant developing and marketing specific drugs for their use. It was largely left to fanciers themselves to experiment with effects and dosages. Sometimes disastrous results followed. Through the years some drugs have become established, others remain experimental. Self-experimentation in fanciers will continue, as more drugs become available and the practice is acceptable if the following provisos are remembered.

1. A new medicine must first be tried on a few less valuable specimens and at least 24 hours must have elapsed before the rest of the flock is treated. If there is any danger of feathering abnormalities developing, flock treatment is delayed at least one month to enable side effects to appear.

2. A large number of worms passed is not a reflection of the efficacy of a drug but is a measure of the severity of the infestation.

3. No worms passed after dosing does not mean that the drug or dosage did not work. Perhaps the drug and dosage were effective but the pigeon was not infested and had no worms to pass.

4. A negative laboratory test on the droppings of any bird does not mean for certain that the bird is free of worms. Immature stages, not yet producing eggs and allowing an egg-free dropping, may be present. A repeat test 10 days later, when the worms have matured, is required. This is particularly true for new introductions or squeakers.

5. Pre- and post-treatment laboratory examination of the faeces is necessary to test the efficacy of a remedy. Post-treatment examination is important to see if ALL worm eggs have disappeared from the droppings.

Dosage Rate; 150 mg/kg (p.o.)

Generic name	Trade name	Present	Marketing Co	Dosage
Piperazine	Antepar	syrup	Coopers	12 ml/litre
	Askaritox	SP	Rumevite	5g/litre
	Predazine	SP	Medpet	5g/litre
	Repzine	SP	Milborrow	5g/litre
	Biozine	liquid	Harkers	

Range of action of the above: Adult Ascaridia

Dosage Rate; 40-50 mg/kg (p.o.)

Generic name	Trade name	Present	Marketing Co	Dosage
Levamisole	Tramisol	liquid	Hoechst	10ml/litre
	Levisol	liquid	Milborrow	10ml/litre
	Ripercol L	liquid	Janssen	8ml/litre
	Rid-O-Worm	liquid	Ciba-Geigy	10ml/litre
	L-Spartakon	tablet	Janssen	1 tablet per bird
	Spartakon	tablet	Harkers	1 tablet per bird
	Dovaworm	tablet	Dova	1 tablet per bird
	Dovaworm	liquid	Dova	5ml/litre
	Levacide	inj.sln.	Norbrook	5ml/litre
	Nemicide	liquid	Janssen	10ml/litre

Range of action of the above: Capillaria, Ascaridia

Morantel	Banmith 11	liquid	Pfizer	1ml/10birds

Range of action of the above: Ascaridia

Febantel	Rintal 2.5%	liquid	Bayer	0.1ml/bird
	Avicas	tablet	Ocopharma	1 tab/bird
Fenbendazole	Panacur 2.5%	liquid	Hoechst	0.2ml/bird
	Panacur	capsule	Hoechst	1 cap/bird
Mebendazole	Multispec	liquid	Janssen	0.6ml/bird
Albendazole	Valbazen(s)	liquid	SK Beecham	on trial
Cambendazole	Ascapilla	caps	Univet	1-2cap/pgn

Range of action of the above: Ascaridia, Capillaria and some action against Tapeworm.

Ivermectin	Ivomec	inject.	MSD-Agvet	1mg/bird
	Eqvalan	paste	MSD-Agvet	
	Oramec	liquid	MSD-Agvet	

Range of action: Ascaridia, Tetrameres (see notes), Acuaria, Capillaria.

Praziquantel	Droncit	tablet	Bayer	1tab/bird

Range of action: Tapeworm, Fluke spp.

Niclosamide	Lintex L	liquid	Bayer	2ml/lit
	Yomesan	tablet	Bayer	.1tab/bird
	Dovalint	tablet	Dova	1tab/bird

Range of action: Tapeworm.

Oxybendazole +Niclosamide	Vitaminthe	paste	Kruger-Med	0.3ml/bird

Range of action: Ascaridia, Capillaria.

Nitroscanate	Lopatol	tablet	CIBA-Geigy	⅛th tab/bird

Rang of action: Tapeworm.

Ascaridia = Roundworms
Capillaria = Hairworms
Tetrameres = Red stomach worms
Acuaria = Spiral stomach worms.

Note. 1. Piperazine acts by paralysing the worms which are then passed normally in the faeces. It is widely used. It does not act on immatures in the bowel wall and is not 100% effective against adults. Dosage must be repeated ten days later to eliminate new adults.

2. Levamisole is effective against capillaria when given for three days. Not active against proventicular worms. Can cause vomiting.

3. Ivermectin is given at very high dosages. Preparation (Ivomec 1% injection, for use in cattle, sheep, pigs.) Injection for solution is diluted, 1 to 4 , with sterile water and given subcutaneously at 0.5 ml/bird. Temporary blindness sometimes occurs, lasting six hours. Tetrameres worms are destroyed one week after injection (flood of semi-developed eggs in faeces).

4. Some Benzimidazoles particularly Cambendazole and Albendazole, are embryo toxic and/or teratogenic in sheep. Similar responses may be expected in pigeon eggs and in growing (devel-

oping) feathers.

– Mebendazole and fenbendazole are known to cause feather abnormalities in developing feathers.

– Mebendazole, fenbendazole and thiabendazole affect hatchability of eggs.

– Albendazole (Valbezan) is toxic for pigeons at effective concentrations.

5. So far no effective and safe product has been found against all three worms commonly found in pigeons, viz. roundworms, capillaria and tapeworms, except Vitaminth, which is expensive and requires individual treatment.

6. Droncit (praziquantel), for pigeons (5mg) is no longer readily available. Droncit 50mg (for dogs and cats) may be used as replacement. Dosage: eighth tablet per bird.

7. Dicestal (dichlorofen) is considered too toxic. Not recommended as a deworming remedy. Effectivity questionable.

7. Banminth (morantel) at three times overdose causes mortality.

8. Levamisole is safer than Tetramisole. Poisoning occurs at three times the recommended level. Overdosing is very easy when used in liquid form which is sold as cattle wormer.

9. Lintex L (niclosamide) is in suspension form and must be vigorously agitated before administration. Water is withheld till birds are thirsty, forcing them to drink before the sediment deposits out. Poisonings (mortalities) have reputedly occurred with niclosamide.

10. Lintex tablets (for dogs) may be broken into eighths. Dose one eighth tablet per pigeon.

The availability of wormers varies greatly from country to country, for example in the United Kingdom only three are licenced for use in racing pigeons – Spartakon, Panacur and Avicas. Biozine is licenced for use in fancy breeds but it's efficacy is poor compared to the new products. It is good policy to use licenced wormers, other products are licenced in other countries, where available and only consider alternative preparations if they are unavailable or if particular problems are experienced. Again these problems will vary from country to country, for instance in the Middle East tapeworms are a more common occurrence than is normal in pigeons in Europe where tapeworms are seldom seen.

All wormers can affect the moult, or more accurately the new feather growth, so bear this in mind when treating your birds.

2. Insecticides

Acute mortality occasionally occurs in pigeons through the injudicious use of insecticides. Even more so than with anthelmintics or other drugs, the the new insecticide must first be tried on a few less-valuable birds. If no undesirable effects are seen within 48 hours, one may assume that the drug is safe to use on the other pigeons.

Dips

Pigeons will not readily bathe in water to which an insecticide has been added as most of these are strong-smelling and repulsive to pigeons. An additional danger is that some of the birds will drink the water. Consequently it has become a common procedure among fanciers to dip (forced bath) their birds.

Neguvon P. Bayer (powder).

Active ingedient; trichlorophen.
Withdrawn from most markets, where it was registered as a deworming powder for horses but is still available elsewhere.

Directions for use: 15 g (one packet) is added to 10 litres water.
Precautions; Contact persons must use waterproof gloves.

Antidote: Atropine 0.05 to 0.1 mg/kg, repeated every 3 hours.

Alugan. Hoechst AG-Vet (powder)

Active ingredient; bromociclene.
Marketed as a wettable powder for dip or wash. May also be used as a powder in the nests. Very low toxicity and well-tolerated by pigeons. Withdrawn from most markets.

Directions for use: Add 20g Alugan to 10 litres water (0.25 % solution).

Treatment; Rapid acting symptomatic treatment eg. sedatives. Do not use adrenaline.

Duramitex. Harkers (liquid)

Active ingredient; malathion. Very low toxicity and may be sprayed directly onto the pigeons. Used also as loft spray.

Directions for use: Add 140 ml to 9 litres water.

Wash

We have found that washing the loft ensures better wetting. Powder given off by the pigeons throughout the previous months, coats the walls and fittings of the loft with a water-repellant layer, preventing thorough wetting of the surfaces.
   The following products named for washing the loft are intended only for use in and on the loft, not directly on the pigeons. They are not indicated for and have not been tested for direct use on the birds.

Coopex. Coopers (powder)

Active ingredient; permethrin, (25 %).

Directions for use: 25g (1 pkt) powder is mixed with 5 litres water. Remove utensils and food trays prior to treatment. Used as a spray or wash inside the loft and will control pigeon flies (Pseudolynchia canariensis) for extended periods up to one year. Before returning birds to the loft ensure that all surfaces have dried thoroughly.

Ambush ICI (liquid)

Active ingredient: permethrin, (500 g per litre).

Directions for use: 12.5ml concentrate is added to 5 litres water. All food trays and utensils must be removed prior to treatment. This is an agricultural product but it has been used with success on pigeons. We use it, similarly to the previous product (Coopex), only on the loft and structures.

Dursban (liquid)

Active ingredient; chlorpyrifos, (480 g per litre). Available for use in the garden. Very toxic if accidentally used on pigeons. Used as a spray or wash inside the loft and will control pigeon flies (Pseudolynchia canariensis) for extended periods up to one year. Before returning birds to the loft ensure that all surfaces have dried thoroughly.

Powders

Powders are safe and easy to use but have the disadvantage of requiring two people, one to hold the bird, the other to apply the insecticide.

Karbadust – Agricura

Active ingredient; carbaryl. Safe for dusting adults as well as nests and babies.

V-Pro, Pro-vet

Active ingredient; carbaryl. As above.

Dovastof – Dova

Contains Carbaryl. As above.

CBM 8 – Phenix

Active ingredient; Propoxur
Dietreen T – Chevita

Active ingredient; tetrachlorvinphos

Use as water soluble powder for a spray or as dusting powder in the loft

VAPOURISING BAR

Vapona

Active ingredient; Dichlorvos

Used as preventative for mosquitoes, flies, lice and mites, their efficacy depends on the degree of ventilation of the loft. In a breeding loft they appear to cause no harm. Effect of chronic inhalation of toxic fumes by pigeons in a racing loft, is unknown, but the advisability is queried.

Chapter 20

Disinfectants

Treatment of the pigeons has little value if, in the presence of disease, cleansing and disinfection of the water containers, food bowls and loft is neglected. Regular disinfection of a healthy environment is instrumental in the prevention of disease as it helps to keep down the numbers of micro-organisms. Cleaning is essential, as most disinfectants are less active in an organically-polluted environment – the cleaner the environment, the better the disinfectant activity.

Disinfectants are grouped into nine different categories but only some of these find practical application in pigeon keeping.

Phenol and the phenolic derivatives are some of the older disinfectants and their use is limited. They are bactericidal, some are fungicidal but they have little effect on viruses and spores.

Examples of their use is found in;

Dettol. Active principal: Chloroxylenol. Useful for general cleanig of utensils.

Jeyes fluid. Well-known disinfectant.

Gill, Hibitane, Phisohex, Hycolin etc. are generally useful for skin disinfection but are not used for pigeons.

Compounds of Chlorine and Iodine.

Chlorine and Chlorine compounds are very effective and are possibly the most powerful disinfectants for pigeon use. They are bacteriocidal, virucidal, fungicidal and sporocidal though their effectivity is directly related to the length of exposure of the microorganisms to the disinfectant, amount of organic pollution and the pH of the environment. Regularly used for disinfecting drinking water containers and for washing the loft. Examples of their use in pigeon keeping are Milton, Jik, Parvocide and Halamid.

Tamed iodine preparations (iodophores) have excellent use in surgical theatres, kitchens, chicken houses etc. Used correctly they are effective against bacteria, fungi and spores but only slightly virucidal. Their effectivity is greatly limited by organic pollution. Betadine and Vensa are used. (The manufacturers of new Vensa claim effective virucidal activity.)

Quaternary Ammonium Compounds (QAC)

Also known "Quats". Most cationic detergents are QAC compounds. They are bactericidal against gram-positive organisms, less so against gram-negative organisms and fungicidal but less effective against viruses and certain protozoa. Mainly employed on skin. Not used much in pigeon keeping.

Examples of products in use are Savlon, Cetavlon and Quaturg.
    Ornisept (based on Cetrimide), made in Belgium and distributed by Squibbs of UK, is used in pigeons.

Gas Chemosterilizers

Formaldehyde is the only one in use. Not sporocidal.

Coccidia oocysts are resistant to disinfection with formaldehyde (formalin) fumigation.

Virkon and Virkon S (Antec International).

Virkon is a colourless, odourless blend of glycols. Tests have shown efficacy following fogging on a par with formaldehyde and better than gluteraldehyde/QAC mixtures.

Virkon S has the same properties as Virkon but is used with Virkon S Fog Enhancer to disinfect the environmental air. Newly available, Virkon appears to possess many advantages.

It is effective against gram-positive and gram-negative bacteria, fungi, moulds, yeasts, mycoplasmas and 17 groups of viruses, including paramyxovirus, herpesvirus, adenovirus, coronavirus and pox virus.

- Safe for operators.

- Virkon can be used to sterilise the drinking water (once the utensils have been disinfected).

- Has been tested non-toxic at recommended levels.

- Pigeons can be returned to the loft as soon as the fog has dispersed.

Recommended for routine disinfection of lofts. Virkon S with the Fog Enhancer may be used after the loft has been sanitised, but the practicality is debatable.

Ucarsan 420 (Janssen)

Contains 20% Gluteraldehyde

Effective against viruses, bacteria, fungi and spores. Following the use of Ucarsan 420, all utensils, food and water containers must be rinsed with clean water, in spite of safety of contact with the product at the recommended (1%) dilution.
   The concentrated solution is poisonous and must not be discarded into a sewer or natural waterway, where it is toxic to fish and other life forms. Rubber gloves and goggles must be worn and the concentrated product handled with care.

Heat is an effective steriliser. Flaming the loft is an accepted means of sterilisation and will destroy coccidia oocysts, worm eggs, bacteria and viruses.

Chapter 21

Vitamins, minerals and amino acids

The pigeon is a natural grain-eating bird, finding the main source of its vitamin and mineral (micro-element) requirements, in various grains. These are, however, not sufficient and deficiencies are complimented by eating vegetables, plant leaves, flowers, insects, snails, soil etc. Artificially we control the vitamin and mineral intake by giving brewer's yeast products, multimineral and multivitamin additives and, very important, by giving a variety of grains, grown on different soils.

IN ESSENCE

Commercial racing mixtures are generally of good quality and vary little regards their protein, carbohydrate or fat content. Individual fanciers prefer one mixture's percentages above another, and believe that the quality of seed in one mixture is supposedly better than another, but the differences are minimal and all camps have their followers.

No pigeon mixtures are fully balanced regarding their vitamin, mineral and amino acid content and supplements are given.

1. Vitamin supplementation.

Brewer's Yeast and fresh greens supply vitamins, minerals, trace elements and protein.

Various artificial vitamin mixtures are available for pigeons, poultry and mammals. They do not differ much. When choosing a vitamin mixture the fancier must first examine his routine supplementation programme. He may already be supplying Brewer's Yeast or greens, milk powder etc., and needs only to compliment what is lacking.

If Brewer's Yeast powder or tablets are given, only vitamin B12 and vitamin E need to be supplemented. The amount of B12 required is infinitesimal. Vitamin E, being fat-soluble, is present in oil-rich grains and excess amounts are stored in the body so that a single supplement will last a long time. Weekly supplementation with wheat germ oil (a favourite) would be adequate.

2. Trace Element supplementation

Trace elements are present in most grains but abundantly supplied by greens or other vegetables. Many artificial vitamin supplements contain a range of trace elements and though deficiency in pigeons is hardly ever recorded (deficiencies occur in conjunction with vitamin deficiencies, which then take precedence), addition to the diet once a week, is considered beneficial.

3. Macro-Mineral supplementation

Minerals, particularly calcium (Ca), are absolutely essential and pigeon breeding cannot be carried on successfully in its absence. Shell grit ($CaCO_3$) must always be available.

4. Essential Amino Acid supplementation

Soya beans supply all the essential amino acids but they are not included in many commercial pigeon mixtures being unpalatable to pigeons unless baked in an oven.

Most standard mixtures contain the essential amino acids. The deficiency of essential amino acids in maize, is compensated for by the other grains. Commercial vitamin preparations usually contain an assortment of the various essential amino acids.

A. The Vitamins

Vitamin A

Vitamin A plays a role in most physiological functions, but is particularly important in:

- bodily growth
- reproduction
- health of mucous membranes
- resistance to infection
- improvement of vision

Vitamin A is found abundantly in maize (800 i.u. per 100 g), spinach (12000 i.u.per 100 g), and green peas. It is low in barley (100 i.u.per 100 g) and other grains (wheat has ±30 i.u. per 100 g).

Daily vitamin A requirements are 80-120 i.u. (international units).

Pigeons fed more than 25% maize, will not suffer vitamin A deficiency. Deficiencies do not occur in practice, and we will not discuss the symptoms, created artificially. Suffice to say that a deficiency will interfere with the above functions, including development in the egg.

Poisoning can occur in pigeons fed too much vitamin A (experimental), resulting in bone malformation and joint pains.

Vitamin B Complex

This group consists of vitamins B1, B2, B3, B6, B12, Pantothenic acid (B5) and B15. The B-group vitamins are so closely linked by their functions and natural occurrence, that they are usually considered as a group.

Overdosing of the B-group vitamins causes premature or unseasonal moulting. No other side effects have been recorded.

Vitamin B1 (thiamine or aneurine)

Very important for man (shortage causes beriberi) and beast. Plays a role in the acquisition of 'form' in pigeons by stimulating the appetite, and influencing the metabolic process whereby stored carbohydrates are used by the muscles for energy, producing lactic acid. This is normally broken down to water and carbon dioxide but with deficient vitamin B1, lactic acid cannot be metabolised further and it accumulates, leading to early fatigue of muscles and mental disturbances.

The functions of vitamin B1 include:

- digestion
- nervous system
- cardiac function
- catabolism (break down) of fats
- carbohydrate metabolism

Vitamin B1 is found naturally in grains. Wheat and maize has 0.45 mg per 100 gram, and barley has more. Brewer's Yyeast is rich in B1 vitamins ($\pm$10 mg per 100 g), as are milk products and greens.

The daily requirements are 0.1 mg per pigeon. Deficiency symptoms are not seen in pigeons fed a normal balanced grain mixture but yeast powder may be given over the food at times of increased stress. Only pigeons on an experimental diet of polished rice show symptoms.

Deficiency symptoms (seen in squabs in the first 10 days):

- loss of appetite
- digestive disturbances
- loss of condition
- muscle weakness
- tremors and opisthotonus
- weak on legs
- green watery droppings

Vitamin B2

Vitamin B2 is a yellow pigment, not destroyed easily by oxidation or heat but extremely sensitive to sunlight. Functions include:

- metabolism of carbohydrates, protein and fats
- development (growth factor)
- helps to produce form
- night vision
- growth of chick in the egg

All seeds fed as pigeon feed, are deficient in vitamin B2. Abundant natural sources are milk products, brewer's yeast ($\pm$3 mg per 100 g), wheat germ, spinach, salad, grass and clover. The average daily requirement for pigeons is $\pm$0.1 mg.

Deficiency symptoms are;

- general weakening
- poor racing results
- poor hatchability of eggs (embryonic mortality in second week)
- poor growth
- nervous symptoms

Vitamin B3 (Vitamin PP, niacine or nicotinamide)

Also known as anti-pellagra vitamin, from the condition described as pellagra, seen in people eating a diet consisting mainly of maize, poor in vitamin B3. Present in Brewer's Yeast.

Functions include:

- digestive processes
- blood formation

Daily requirements for pigeon are +1 to 1.5 mg.

Deficiency symptoms include:

- retarded growth
- poor feathering
- poor moult
- unformed droppings
- lack of appetite

Panthothenic acid (Vitamin B5)

Pantothenic acid probably affects feather quality (deficiency caused delayed growth, decolorisation and curling of the feathers in chickens), including pigmentation.
   It is found in adequate amounts in feedgrains and is abundantly present in brewer's yeast (11mg per 100g). Also found in milk powder and sprouted wheat.

Deficiency symptoms include:

- poor pigmentation
- poor growth
- poor quality plumage

Vitamin B6 (pyridoxine)

Plays a role in general metabolism and is important to counteract the ageing process. (Experiments with apes have shown it to counteract calcification of bloodvessels.)

Naturally present in sprouted wheat, milk powder, diverse greens, brewer's yeast, maize, other grains and legumes.

Functions include:

- metabolism
- conversion of unsaturated fatty acids
- help with producing form

Daily requirements are 0.25 to 3.0 mg per pigeon.

Deficiency symptoms include:

- lack of form
- poor hatchability

Vitamin B12 (Cyanocobalamin)

Vitamin B12, though needed in ultra-small amounts, is an important requirement to be added to the diet of pigeons kept prisoner, as it is totally lacking from plant material. Because they cannot forage at will, these birds miss the opportunity to catch and eat insects, snails etc, which form a natural source of the vitamin.

The essential functions include:

- synthesis of red blood cells
- important growth factor
- support embryo growth

Occurs in a fermentation process in the presence of cobalt, as in fermenting manure heaps. Requirements are minimal, +0.0001 mg per day per pigeon.

Deficiency symptoms include:

- anaemia
- poor hatchability
- poor rearing results

- poor growth
- deficient feathering
- erosion of the gizzard

Vitamin B15

Recent discovery and introduction into pigeon racing. Functions include:

- donation of methyl group that activates oxygen metabolism in tissue cells. Believed to increase endurance through better oxygen utilisation. Recommended for long distance racing.
- detoxifying action in liver
- lipotropic action.

Included in some vitamin preparations eg. Dovawin.

Vitamin C (Ascorbic acid)

Pigeons can manufacture vitamin C for their needs. Controversy exists about the value of vitamin C supplementation of the diet. There is some indication that requirements are increased during stress and supplementation of the diet does no harm. Functions of vitamin C include:

- plays a role in respiration,
- plays a role in the nutrition of red blood cells
- involved with the recovery of tissues and defense mechanisms.

Deficiency causes thin egg shells.

Vitamin D

Cod liver oil contains large quantities of various kinds of vitamin D3 (the active form of the vitamin) and is valuable as a supplement over the food. It becomes rancid and rapidly loses its vitamin content, including vitamin E (influences fertility), in the presence of light and air.

Vitamin D is formed in the body from precursors, under the influence of the ultra-violet rays from sunlight. Glass absorbs ultra-violet light and is not recommended in a breeding establishment unless the birds are subjected at some time to the direct rays of the sun. Free-flying pigeons get sufficient exposure and do not need supplementation of their diet.

Functions of vitamin D include:

- regulation of calcium/phosphorus ratio
- important role in bone formation
- role in defense mechanisms of the body

Requirements for pigeons lie between 20 and 30 i.u. per day. Deficiency symptoms are similar to calcium deficiency, i.e.:

- rickets
- curved sternum (can be cause by other conditions)
- deformed legs
- weak, brittle bones
- weak beak
- thin eggshells

Poisoning occurs with repeated enormous dosages of cod liver oil and gives rise to malformed bone formation.

Vitamin E (alpha-tocopherol)

Widely known as fertility vitamin. All grains contain vitamin E. Deficiency does not occur, other than when rancid, stale oil-bearing seeds (linseed, rape seed, sunflower etc.) are fed. Vitamin E is destroyed in old, rancid seed.
   Sprouted grains are rich in vitamin E (maize germ; 16mg and wheat germ; 30mg per 100 g). Wheat germ oil contains 520mg per 100g. The functions of vitamin E include:

- promotion of fertility
- synergistic effect with vitamin A (defense mechanism)
- to act as detoxifying agent

Deficiency symptoms include:

- infertility (cocks)
- dead-in-shell (hens)
- muscular dystrophy (synergistic with selenium)

The vitamin has been given with success in combination with Vitamin A and D3, to correct infertility, particularly in old cocks.

Vitamin H (biotin)

Present in grain germs and Brewer's Yeast. Daily requirement for pigeons is 0.01 mg. Found in adequate amount in daily ration.

Main function is:

- growth factor for micro-organisms.

Deficiency symptoms include:

- dermatosis
- infected legs and sore eyes

Vitamin K

Obtained by the pigeon in its food and by synthesis. Greens are an excellent source.

Function of vitamin K

- fortifies the blood vessels
- promotes blood coagulation

Deficiency symptoms include:

- interference with blood coagulation

Choline (vitamin J)

The function of choline can be replaced by vitamin B12 acting with methionine (amino acid). Choline is a growth factor, although doubt exists whether it is a true vitamin. High values are found in Brewer's Yeast, greens and soya beans. Functions of choline include:

- counteracts fatty degeneration of the liver
- growth factor
- promotes the action of the liver and kidneys

Deficiency symptoms include:

- liver degeneration
- haemorrhages in the kidney
- retarded growth

Para-aminobenzoic acid (PABA)

Present in greens and Brewer's Yeast.

Functions include:

- growth factor
- influences plumage (with inositol)

Deficiency symptoms include:

- poor feathering
- retarded growth of squeakers

Inositol (vitamin I)

Growth factor. Some animals appear to synthesize the vitamin themselves. Present in sprouted grains and green peas.
   Deficiencies rarely occur but include liver degeneration because of fatty accumulation.

Folic acid (vitamin M, glutamic acid)

Found in greens and Brewer's Yeast. Adequate amounts in the diet if these are given regularly. Main functions:

- formation of red blood cells
- promotes healthy pigmentation of feathers
- growth factor

Deficiency symptoms include:

- retarded growth
- anemia
- decolouration of plumage
- poor hatchability

Rutin (vitamin P)

Found in greens.

Main function; regulation of capillary permeability. Deficiency seen as coagulation in capillaries.

B. The Trace Elements

Trace elements are essential for the proper functioning of the body but are required only in minute quantities. The more important ones are zinc, cobalt, copper, iodine, manganese, molybdenum, iron etc.

The trace elements (minerals) are present in grain, but abundant in vegetables and greens, particlurly carrots, spinach, parsley, cabbage, sprouts, lettuce, endive and particularly tomatoes, in addition to which, they are rich in vitamins A and C.

Zinc plays a role in respiration.

Cobalt is an essential ingredient of vitamin B12. Without it, deficiency of vitamin B12 would occur, leading to anaemia and nervous degeneration.

Copper (Cu), molybdenum (Mb) and iron (Fe) are essential in the formation of red blood cells. Iron plays a role in muscle formation.

Excessive iron in the diet, causes liver pathology and haemosiderosis of the liver cells is seen if the iron content of the drinking water is too high.

Iodine (I) plays an important role in the functioning of the thyroid and a deficiency of the element leads to thyroid hypoactivity. Thyroid activity is closely correlated with sexual fervour, essential in racing pigeons, particularly widowhood cocks. The thyroid plays an active but complex role, with vitamin B1, in the burning of fats for energy, an abundance of which is essential for producing form.

Iodine is freely available in natural products eg. radish, tomato, spinach, lettuce and, above all, kelp is rich in this mineral. It is believed that proximity to the sea will prevent iodine deficiency as enough iodine is absorbed from the sea-air. Seawater and plants are rich in iodine.

Selenium (Se) reinforces the anti-oxidant properties of vitamin E on cell membranes. The two substances work together to protect the integrity of cell membranes. Deficiency leads to white muscle disease, in mammals.

Magnesium (Mg) is found in greens. It is active in bone formation, nerve pulse transmission and activation of enzymes.

C. The Macro-minerals

The macro-minerals must be present in large (as opposed to miniscule) amounts in the diet of racing pigeons. Calcium and phosphorus occur in substantial amounts in the composition of bone, muscle and nervous tissues.

Calcium (Ca)

Found throughout the body, as calcium phosphate in bone and as free (ionised) and bound calcium in blood. Calcium in the bones serves as reservoir for calcium in the blood.

Calcium is low in a normal grain diet (seeds are low in calcium and high in phosphorus) and in order to keep the important calcium:phosphorus (Ca:P) ratio at an optimum ($\pm$ 1:1.5), it is important that calcium-holding grit is always available. For this purpose plain oyster shell grit or shell grit is ideal and pigeons will avidly eat it. If given the opportunity, pigeons will eat enough calcium to avoid deficiencies, the fancier has only to make it available. Sunlight, via vitamin D3, also helps to stabilize the Ca:P ratio.

Phosphorus (P)

Present in bone and nervous tissue. Plays a role in the chemical reactions responsible for metabolising fats and carbohydrate to produce energy.

Abundantly present in grains and birds must be fed calcium to prevent the important Ca:P ratio from being upset. Deficiencies practically never occur.

Sulphur (S)

Sulphur is an important constituent of skin, feathers and nails. It is present in grains, legumes and greens. Additional supplementation seems unnecessary though we know of champion fliers who give it regularly, particularly in the breeding and moulting seasons.

The pigeons would possibly do equally well without it. Feeds (cabbage) containing excessive sulphur was responsible for poor health, abortions and reduced fertility in cattle and sheep. Similar effects have not been noted in pigeons but detailed studies have not been done.

Sodium (Na) + Chloride (Cl)

Constituents of table salt. Salt-starved pigeons eat salt hungrily but it has not been shown that they require supplementation. It is a useful bait to entice pigeons to eat other minerals and rearing pigeons do so voraciously when salt is mixed with charcoal and other elements.

D. The Amino Acids

Amino acids are the building blocks of proteins, which form about 80% of the body's waterless mass. Essential amino acids cannot be manufactured by the body like the other amino acids and require to be present in the diet, either naturally or supplemented.

Arginine, histidine, leucine, isoleucine, valine, treonine, methionine, phenylalanine, tryptophane and lysine are the known essential amino acids and must be in the diet.

The total protein percentage of a diet must be continually adjusted to meet the pigeon's demand, which varies according to the stage of its annual cycle. During times of high activity (racing), a diet must contain more carbohydrates, during the resting period more fibre and when rearing babies a high percentage of protein is required. Crop milk, which consists of the sloughed off cells of the internal epithelial layer of the crop, contains no carbohydrate but is high in protein and fat.

An analysis by Ferrando yielded; 75-77% water, 11-13% protein, 5-7%fat and 1.2-1.8% minerals. (This percentage of protein and fat looks very ordinary, at first glance, until one considers that no extra water is consumed and that the analysis should rather be looked at from a dry basis.) Leash, in another study, found that the crop content changed dramatically during the first month of a pigeon's life. On day one an analysis on dry basis, yielded 27% fat, 46% protein and 21% carbohydrate. On day 7 it abruptly changed to 5% fat and 27% protein and continued to change to day 27 when 3% fat, 17% protein and 74% carbohydrate were recorded.

It is uncertain whether these birds were fed ad lib or were forced to eat whatever was supplied. What is apparent is that the recorded changes fit in nicely with a decreasing percentage of crop milk fed to the nestlings.

BIOLOGICAL VALUE

The biological value of a seed refers to the number and concentration of the essential amino acids available in the seed, relative to the amino acids needed by the body to form proteins. A feed mixture must therefore, in addition to being balanced with regard to proteins, carbohydrates and fats, have a high biological value in regard of the proteins. In other words, the essential amino acid content of the individual seeds making up the mixture, must compliment each other. Having a diet with a high total protein content but low biological value, is equally as bad as having low proteins in the diet and will lead to negative nitrogen balance.

We talk of a nitrogen balance because all proteins contain roughly 16% nitrogen. From the amount of nitrogen in the excreted uric acid, we can calculate the amount of protein broken down. Other measures are of the nitrogen in the droppings (undigested protein) and of the protein consumed. A negative nitrogen balance occurs when the nitrogen excreted, is greater than the nitrogen (protein) consumed and the bird has a protein loss. This is usually owing to poor diet, disease or severe loss through burns (in mammals).

To counteract a negative nitrogen balance the birds must receive a ration balanced in amino acids, by being fed a mixture containing as many seeds as possible. Any deficiency in essential amino acids can be corrected by feeding concentrates (fish meal has a good balance of essential amino acids) containing the required amino acids or by medicating the drinking water. An excess of amino acids do no harm.

Deficiency of:

- methioninine, exacerbates choline and vitamin B12 deficiency.
- lysine, causes impaired feather pigmentation.
- arginine, causes feather rotation.

Sorghum is low in tryptophane. Darker-coloured sorghum is high in tannic acid, and may cause depression of growth. High in lysine.

Maize is low in lysine and tryptophane.

Soya beans are high in lysine as well as the other amino acids.

Sunflower seed is low in lysine but contains all the other essential amino acids.

Appendix A

Glossary

All explanations for terms and words apply specifically to their application in this book.

abscess. A localised collection of pus, consisting of organisms, necrotic cells and tissue fluid. Abscesses in pigeons are solid and caseous.

acid. Having a pH below 7

acute. Having a short and relatively severe course.

aerocystitis. Inflammation of an airsac; airsacculitis.

adhesion. The abnormal joining of two or more body structures, often following tissue damage or infection.

administration. The method of introducing a drug or medication to the body. This includes the dosage, schedule and route.

aetiology. See etiology.

affinity. Natural attraction

air sac. Membranous sac, of which the pigeon has eleven, that is connected to the lungs.

airsacculitis. Inflammation of an airsac; aerocystitis.

alveolus (alveoli). In mammals, an airsac of the lungs formed by the terminal dilations of a bronchilolus. Does not occur in pigeons.

alkaline. Having a pH above 7.

amino acid. Any one of a class of organic compounds containing the amino (NH_2) group and the carboxyl (COOH) group. They are the basic units into which food proteins are broken down during digestion and from which body proteins are formed in cells and organs.

anaemia. A state of the blood in which it is deficient in haemoglobin or red cells, resulting in paleness of the skin and membranes.

anaphylaxis. An acute and exaggerated allergenic response

followed by shock.

anorexia. A loss or decrease in appetite.

antibody. A modified serum globulin, synthesized by an animal in response to antigenic stimulus, which reacts specifically with the homologous antigen.

arbovirus. A virus carried and reproduced by an arthropod and transmitted through its bite to a vertebrate host, in which it also reproduces.

arthritis. Inflammation of a joint, either infectious (eg. paratyphoid) or non-infectious (synovial gout).

arthropod. Largest animal phylum, characterised by jointed limbs and hard jointed external skeleton; includes insects, arachnids, crustaceans and trilobites.

ascites. Accumulation of straw-coloured fluid in the abdominal cavity.

attenuated. Reduced in pathogenicity or virulence.

ataxia. Lack of muscular co-ordination, resulting in unsteadiness and haphazard flying.

atrophy. Wasting away or dimunition in the size of a cell, tissue, organ or part.

avitaminosis. Disease condition caused by lack of vitamins.

bacteraemia. Bacteria in the bloodstream.

bacteria. Minute one-celled organisms that multiply by dividing.

bile. A fluid secreted by the liver and poured into the intestine; it assists in digestion.

blood quill. Quill of a feather that remains blood-filled for an abnormally long time.

bronchiolus (bronchioli). A finer division of a bronchus.

bronchus (bronchi). Branch of the trachea.

bruise. An impact injury without a break in the superficial surface.

calcareous. Containing lime or calcium.

cancer. A cellular growth the natural course of which is fatal an usually associated with formation of secondary tumours.

candling. Examining an egg with a strong light as background to see development, infertility etc.

carrier. A pigeon that harbours and sheds an infectious agent without showing clinical evidence or signs.

cervical. Pertaining to or of the neck.

chronic. An infection characterized by a continued or long-lasting course.

cirrhosis. State whereby liver cells are invaded and replaced by fibrotic tissue.

clinical. Demonstrating visible evidence of its presence.

cloaca. The lower end of the pigeon's combined digestive, urinary

and genital tracts, collecting and releasing faeces and urinary
excretions.

coagulation. Conversion of blood from a fluid to a solid state.
coccidiostat. A chemical used to control coccidia oocyst
production.

concrement. A calcified tubercle or similar mass.

congenital. Referring to a condition that exists at birth.

congestion. The abnormal accumulation of blood in body
structures.

conjunctiva. A membrane that lines the eyelids and covers the
eyeball in front.

conjunctivitis. Inflammation of the conjunctiva.

contagious. Capable of being transmitted fron one pigeon to
another.

coryza. An acute catarrhal condition of the nasal mucous
membrane, attended with a ropy discharge from the nostrils.

course. The period of disease from start to recovery or death.

crustacean. Large class of the arthropods, many with a hard shell
and many legs; includes crabs, lobsters, woodlice etc.

culling. Removing a pigeon from a flock, usually because of inferior
performances or prospects.

culture. A growth of micro-organisms or other living cells.

cytoplasm. The body of a cell excluding the nucleus.

cyanosis. A bluish discolouration of tissues owing to lack of
oxygenation.

embryonated. Having an embryo. Refers to eggs (pigeon or
parasite) in which the germ has started activity.

debride. To remove all foreign matter or devitalised tissue from a
lesion.

dehydration. Loss of body fluid.

desiccate. To make thoroughly dry.

distal. Farthest from the centre or point of attachment.

dorsal. Referring to the upper surface.

dilatation. Distension or stretching of a part or organ.

drug resistance. Condition wherein micro-organisms are immune
to the effects of certain medicines. Can be congenital or
acquired.

dyspnoea. Difficult or laboured breathing.

eggy. Condition of a hen, due to lay.

encephalitis. Inflammation of the brain.

enteritis. Inflammation of the intestine.

enzootic. Referring to a disease that persists in a specific
population of animals or birds.

enzyme. An organic compound, often a protein, capable of catalytic activity in the body.

epidemic. Referring to a disease attacking many people in the same regiom at the same time.

epidemiology. The study of factors affecting epidemics.

epiglottis. The slit-like to oval opening of the anterior (upper) end of the trachea.

epizootic. Attacking many animals in the same region at the same time.

erosion disease. A disease that prevents successful performances without showing clinical signs.

etiology. Cause of disease.

flagellum (flagellae). Whiplike structure of micro-organism that produces motility by its actions.

focal. Referring to localised centres of change.

fungus. Any one of a class of microscopic or larger vegetable organisms that do not produce chlorophyl and reproduce by spores.

gizzard. The mucular stomach for grinding the food after it is mixed with gastric juices from the proventriculus.

glycogen. A carbohydrate produced by the liver for conversion to dextrose.

gout. A condition resulting in excessive precipitation of urates in and on body tissues and synovial membranes.

gravid. Pregnant.

haemagglutination. The clumping of red blood cells.

haemolytic. Referring to the release of haemoglobin from the red blood cells by their rupture.

haemopoietic. Pertaining to the formation of blood cells.

histopathology. The pathology in a body seen at microscopic level.

hormone. A discrete chemical substance which has a specific effect on the activities of other organs and is secreted into the body fluids by an endocrine gland; can be manufactured synthetically.

haematoma. A swelling containing effused blood.

hermaphrodite. A pigeon possessing developed sex organs of both sexes.

hypertrophy. Compensatory enlargement of an organ or part.

idiosyncratic. Having an individual and peculiar susceptibility to some drug.

inertia. Inactivity

infection. Invasion of and replication in the body by pathogenic micro-organisms and the reaction of the tissues to their presence.

infestation. Invasion of the body by arthropods, including insects, mites and ticks.

infiltration. Accumulation of cells or substances not normal to the tissues.

inflammation. Condition of living tissue, marked by heat, swelling, redness and usually pain, arising from the repair process or from the action by the damaged tissues or body to remove or destroy invading organisms.

haemorrhage. Bleed.

internal laying. Laying eggs within the body cavity.

immunity. The power of pigeon to resist a specific infection.

inapparent infection. An infection without clinical signs.

inclusion body. Round, oval or irregular shaped body within the nucleus/cytoplasm of a cell, caused by a virus infection.

incubation period. The interval between exposure to infection and the appearance of clinical disease.

inspissated. Thickened, dried and made less fluid.

inflammation. Tissue reaction to injury.

keratitis. Inflammation of the cornea of the eye.

keratosis. Horny growth of epithelial tissue.

mandible. One of two bones (fused) forming the lower beak.

malformation. Defective or abnormal formation; deformity.

mechanical carrier. An individual that transmits an agent of a disease without participating in its development.

maxilla. Bone forming the upper beak.

morbidity. The ratio of sick to healthy pigeons in a group, from a specific cause, occurring within a specific time.

mortality. The ratio of the total number of deaths in a group, from a specific cause, occurring in a specific time.

mucous membrane. A membrane lining the canals and cavities of the body, which communicate with the external air.

mucus. The free slime of the mucous membranes, composed of their secretion mucin, formed by the mucous glands, various inorganic salts, desquamated cells and leukocytes.

necrosis. Death of a cell or group of cells in contact with live tissue.

nephritis. Inflammation of the kidney.

nephrosis. Any disease of the kidney.

nictitating membrane. The third eyelid.

obesity. Excessive accumulation of fat.

oedema. Presence of abnormally excessive amounts of water in the tissues.

oesophagus. The tubular structure connecting the pharynx to the crop.

opthalmitis. Inflammation of the eye.

oviduct. Tube in the body through which an ovum moves on its passage from the ovary to the outside, while having albumen, eggshell membrane and egg-shell formed around it.

paralysis. Loss of motor function.

parenteral. Not through the digestive canal.

paresis. Partial loss of motor function.

pathogen. Any disease-producing organism.

pathogenesis. The development of disease.

pathogenicity. The ability of a micro-organism to produce disease.
   pathology. The structural and functional changes in tissues and
   organs of the body, caused by disease.

perforation. The act of piercing or penetrating through a part,
   usually the bowel; puncture.

peritonitis. Inflammation of the peritoneum.

peritoneum. Serous membrane lining the abdominal walls and
   investing the viscera.

pH. Symbol used to express acidity or alkalinity. It measures the
   concentration of hydrogen ions. 7 is the neutral point.

pipey feather. Feather that fails to break loose from its sheath.

polyuria. The passage of anormal amounts of urine

polydipsia. Excessive thirst.

proventriculus. Gland, secreting digestive enzymes and situated in
   the oesophagus between the crop and gizzard.

prolapse. Turning inside out.

pneumonia. Inflammation of the lungs.

pseudohermaphrodite. An apparent hermaphrodite, where the
   gonads are of one sex but the secondary sex characteristics
   arouse doubt as to the true sex.

pseudomalaria. An infection with Haemoproteus spp.

pseudomembranous. Pertaining to a false membrane.

rales. An abnormal respiratory sound heard on auscultation,
   indicating some pathological condition.

resistance. The natural ability of a pigeon to ward off the
   deleterious effects of poisons, toxins, pathogenic organisms etc.

rupture. Forcible tearing or bursting of a part.

salpingitis. Inflammation of the oviduct.

scolex. The head and neck of tapeworm.

secondary infection. Infection by a microorganism following
   infection by another organism.

septicemia. A presence of pathogenic organisms in the blood.

serosa. Serous membrane.

serous membrane. Membrane that is bathed by serum.

sinusitis. Inflammation of the sinus membranes.

sourcrop. Crop with acid, fetid odour to the contents.

strain. A group or family within a species with a distinct
   hereditary character.

stricture. Abnormal reduction in size of a duct from contraction.

subacute. Somewhat acute; between acute and chronic.

susceptibility. The degree of readiness to be affected or be acted upon.

suture. A surgical stitch.

synovitis. Inflammation of the synovial membranes of the joints, tendon sheaths and bursae.

synthesis. Biological manufacture.

systemic. Involving all body systems.

toxic. Having a poisonous effect.

toxin. A poison of animal or vegetable origin.

toxaemia. Toxin or poison in the bloodstream.

trophozoite. A protozoan in an early stage of development when it occupies an epithelial or blood cell.

trachea. The windpipe.

trauma. A wound or injury.

trichomoniasis. Infestation with trichomonas; cropcanker.

ulcer. A degenerative lesion on open skin or mucous membrane, other than a wound.

uraemia. Accumulation of urinary components in the blood.

vaccine. A product designed to produce an immune reaction within the body.

vector. An intermediate host that transmits the causative agent of a disease.

vestigial. Rudimentary.

vermicide. Drug used to kill worms.

verminosis. Infestation with worms.

ventral. Pertaining to the lower end or surface of a structure.

viraemia. Virus in the bloodstream.

virus. Any group of submicroscopic infective agents, not capable of multiplying outside living cells.

viscera. Organs within the body cavity.

xanthoma. A condition characterised by the presence of yellow colour in the skin, due to the presence of lipoids.

Appendix B

Abbreviations and equivalent measures

1 meter (m)	100 cm	39.37 inches
1 centimetre (cm)	0.01 m	0.3937 in
1 millimeter (mm)	0.001 m	.03937 in
1 micrometer (um)	.000,001 m	0.000,03937 in
1 kilogram (kg)	1000 g	2.2046 pounds (lb)
1 gram (g)	1g = 1000 mg	15.432 grain (gr)
1 centigram (cg)	.01 g	1.5432 gr
1 milligram (mg)	.001 g	0.0154 gr
1 microgram (mcg)	.000001 g = .001 mg	0.000,0154 gr
1 pound (lb)	16 oz (7000 gr)	453.59 g
1 ounce (oz)	437.5 gr	28.349 g
1 grain (gr)	0.000143 lb	0.06418 g
1 gallon imp. (gall)	4 quarts	4.546 l
1 quart (qt)	2 pints	1.136 l
1 pint (pt)	34.68 cu in	.568 l
1 fluid ounce (fl oz)	0.06 pt	28.4 ml
1 litre (l)	1000 ml	61.025 cu in
1 millilitre (ml)	.000 l	0.061 cu in
1 cu.m (1mx1mx1m)	1000 l	1.308 cu yd
1 sq. m	0.01 are	1.1960 sq.yd

1 sq centimetre		0.155 sq.in
1 cu.cm (cc)	1.0 ml	.061 cu.in

1 teaspoon (tsp)	±4 ml (liquid)
	±4 g (powder)
1 tablespoon (tbsp)	±16 ml (liquid)
	±16 g (powder)

Notes

1. A cc. (cubic centimetre) and a ml (millilitre) measure the same volume. They are freely interchangeable.

2. A kitchen teaspoon is ± 4 ml, but they are not all the same, some being bigger and others smaller. (A measuring spoon is calibrated at 5ml.) For an accurate measurement, a pharmacist should be consulted.

3. Powders do not all weigh the same, but they are approximately the weight of water (i.e. at sea level 1ml water at 4° C weighs 1g). For rough estimates we can work on 1tsp. powder weighing 4g but make small adjustments where necessary.

4. A trade medicine giving its concentration in percentage form, means that so many parts of the active ingredient are contained per hundred parts medicine. When working out the dosage it is convenient to work in milligrams and grams (and millilitres and litres), so we multiply the given percentage by 10.

eg. 5.5% powder, multipied by 10 translates to 55 mg/g.

Equally, 10% solution becomes 100 ml/l (10x10=100)

5. A dosage instruction given as p.p.m., means parts active ingredient per million trade medicine. The same numbers are used when converting;

eg. 10 p.p.m. = 10 mg/l

and 25 p.p.m. = 25mg/kg

Appendix C

Bibliography

Chapter 2: Problems encountered

Calder, W.A. and King, J.R. (1974) Thermal and Caloric relations of birds. In; Avian Biology, D.S. Farmer and J.R. King, Eds, New York Academic Press, 1974, Vol 4., 259-413.
Kendeigh, S.C. The role of metabolism in the development of temperature regulation in birds. (1939) J. Exp. Zool. 82: 419-438.
Vermeijen, L. and Aerts, J. Communique; Hoe wy ze keuren, 30-31.

Chapter 3: Problem solving

Schrag,L., Enz, H., Klette, H., Messinger, H. (1985) Healthy Pigeons. 2nd Ed., 48-53.
Viaene, N. (1986) Personal communication.

Chapter 4: Viral diseases

Alexander, D.J.,Russell, P.H. and Collins, M.S. (1984) Paramyxovirus type 1 infection of racing pigeons: 1 Characterisation of isolated viruses. Vet. Rec. 114: 444-446.
Alexander, D.J., Parsons, G., Marshall, R. (1986) Avian paramyxovirosis type 1 infections of racing pigeons: 4 Laboratory assessment of vaccination. Vet. Rec. 118: 262-266.
Botha. O.J.B. (1993) Die adenovirus/E. coli-sindroom in wedvlugduiwe in Suid Afrika. SA Posduif/Racing Pigeon 7 no 4; 24-26.
Botha, W.S. Path. report no. 85/5021 and Path. report no. 85/4746.
Box, P.G., Holmes, H.C and McCartney, E. (1985) Vaccination of pigeons against paramyxovirus 1 infection. Vet. Rec. 117: 555-

556.

Cunningham, C.H. (1965) Fowl pox. In E.H. Biester and L.H. Schwarte, Eds, Diseases of poultry 5th Ed., I.S.U.P., Iowa.

DeVriese, L. (1986) Diergeneesk. Memorandum 33 no 1; 47, 58.

Hanson, R.P. and Sinha, S.K. (1952) Epizootic of Newcastle disease in pigeons and studies on transmission of the virus. Poultry Science 31:404.

Kaleta, E.F., Alexander D.J. and Russell, P.H. (1985) The first isolation of the avian PMV-1 virus responsible for the current panzootic in pigeons? Av. Path. 14: 553-557.

Karstad, L. (1971) Arboviruses. In; J.W. Davis. R.C. Anderson,

Karstad, L., D.O. Trainer (1971). Eds, Infectious and Parasitic Diseases of Wild Birds. 1st Ed. 17-21. I.U.S.P. Iowa.

Karstad, L. (1971) Pox. In; J.W. Davis, R.C. Anderson, L.Karstad,

D.O. Trainer. Eds, Infectious and Parasitic Diseases of Wild Birds. 1st Ed. 34-41. I.U.S.P., Iowa.

Kaschula, V.R. (1950) The epizootiology of Newcastle disease and its control by vaccination. J. S. African Vet. Med. Assoc. 21: 134.

Kaschula, V.R. (1952) The domestic pigeon as a possible carrier of Newcastle disease. Onderstepoort J. Vet. Res. 25: 25.

Kirme, P. (1967) Pox in wild birds; an annotated bibliography. Wildlife Diseases 11: 209.

Lemahieu, P. (1988) Adeno-coli infection in homing pigeons. International Pigeon World no. 10;18.

Mohammed, M.A., Sokkar, S.M. and Tantawi, H.H. (1978) Avian Pathology 7:637.

Mulligan, T.P.S., Beyers, N., Dietrich, B.E., Anstey, L., Carter, J.W.

Path. report Lab no; 88123.

Olesiuk, O.M. (1951) Influence of environmental factors on viability of Newcastle disease virus. Am. J. Vet. Res. 12: 152.

Palmer, S.F. and Trainer, D.O. (1971) Infectious and Parasitic diseases of wild birds. 1st Ed: 3-16. I.S.U.P., Ames, Iowa.

Pollard, B. and Marais, E.J. (1983) Pigeon Herpesvirus confirmed in South Africa. J.S.A.V.A. 54 no 4; 247-248.

Schrag, L., Enz, H., Klette, H., Messinger H. [a] (1985) Healthy Pigeons. 5th Engl. rev. ed.

Senne, D. (1985) Summary notes of a Symposium on paramyxovirus and vaccine production convened by the American Pigeon Fanciers' Council, July 1985.

Sprunt, D.H. (1955) The pathology of psittacosis. In E.R. Beaudette, Ed, Psittacosis, Epidemiology and Control. Rutgers Univ. Press. New Brunswick.

Stam, J.W.E. (1986) Personal communication.

Stam, J.W.E. (1980) Diktaat; Vogelziekten, 3de ed.; 113-114.

Stosskopf, J.P. (1984) A considered response to paramyxovirosis. transl. from Colombophile Bulletin National no. 34.

Tantawi, H.H., Al-Salluji, S.M. and Al-Salluji, H.K. (1980) Avian diseases 24: 1011.

Ulbrich, F. and Sodan, U. (1965) Natural infection in pigeons with Newcastle disease virus. Mh. Vet. Med. 20: 340, 1965. Abstr. Vet. Bull. 35: 774, 1965.

Terskikh, I.I. (1964) Problems of medical virology, ornithosis. First All Union Symp., Vol 10; Ivanovsky Institute of Virology, Acad. Med. Sci. USSR, Moscow.

Van der Sluis, J. (1984) Communique; Paramyxo by duiven. Najaar 1984.

Viaene, N. Communique; Paramyxovirus-1 of racing pigeons.

Viaene, N., Spanoghe, L., DeVriese, B., Bynens, A. and DeVos,A. (1984) Vaccinatieproeven tegenover paramyxovirus by duiven. Vl. Diergeneesk. Tydschr. 53: 42-52.

Vindevogel, H., Dagenais, L., Lansival, B. Pastoret, P.P. (1981) Incidence of rotavirus, adenovirus and herpesvirus in pigeons. Vet. Rec. 109; 285-286.

Vindevogel, H. and Duchatel, J.P. (1985) Understanding paramyxovirosis. Infofile on pigeon racing.

Zwart, P. Path. report no D82/301.

Chapter 5: Bacterial and fungal diseases

Baaij, J. (1983) Salmonellose by Postduiven. Een studie over epidemiologie en preventie. 3, 17-18, 33.

DeVriese, L. (1986) Diergeneesk. Memorandum 33 no 1; 36.

Ruger, R. and Raddei, J. (1981) Vergleichende Wirksamkeitsprufungen von 5 verschiedenen inaktivierten Vaksinen gegen die Salmonellose der Tauben. Dtsch. Tierartztl. Wschr., 88; 511-514

Scholtens R.Th. and Carolli, G. (1971) Role of pigeons in the spread of Salmonellosis: incidence of different types of Salmonella typhimurium var. copenhagen. Anthonie v. Leeuwenhoek., 37; 473-476.

Schrag, L., Enz, H., en Klette, H. (1974) Gesonde Duiwe. 1ste druk; 59.

Sinclair, D.V. (1980) Respiratory disease in pigeons. Vet. Record, May 31, 1980.

Stam, J.W.E. (1980) Dictaat; Vogelziekten 3de ed.; 154.

T-W-Fiennes R.N. (1982) Diseases of Bacterial origin. In Margaret L. Petrak, Ed. Diseases of Cage and Aviary Birds. 2nd Ed. 24;

505.

Viaene, N. (1986) Personal communication.

Wallis, A.S. (1991) Common conditions of domestic pigeons. In Practice, May 1991.

Whitney, L.F. (1969) Keep your pigeons flying. 2nd ed.; 113, 137-138.

Chapter 6: Protozoal diseases

Cook, R.S. Trainer, D.O. and Glazener, W.C. (1966) Haemoproteus in wild turkeys from the coastal bend of South Texas. J. Protozool. 13; 588.

DeVriese, L. (1986) Diergeneesk. Memorandum 33 no 1; 43, 44, 47

Finlay, P. and Manwell, H.D. (1956) Toxoplasma from the crow, a new natural host. Exptl. Parasitol. 5; 149.

Garnham, P.C.C. (1966) Malarial Parasites and other Haemosporidia. Oxford, Blackwell, 1114 pp.

Jansen, B.C. (1952) The occurrence of some hitherto undescribed Leucocytozoon and Haemoproteus species in South African birds. Onderstepoort J. Vet. Res. 25; 3.

Keymer, I.F. (1982) Parasitic Diseases. Contrib. to M.L. Petrak, Ed.   Diseases of Cage and Aviary Birds, 2nd ed; 535-598.

Kocan, R.M. and Knisley, J.O. (1970) Challenge infection as a means of determining the rate od disease-resistant Trichomonas gallinae-free birds in a population. J. Wildlfe Diseases 6; 13.

Levine, N.D. (1973) Protozoan Parasites of Domestic Animals and of Man. 2nd ed.; 406 pp.

Levine, N.D. and Kantor, S. (1959) Check-list of blood parasites of birds of the Columbiformes. Wildlife Diseases 1; 1.

Manwell, H.D. and Drobeck, H.P. (1952) Mammalian toxoplasmosis in birds. Expetl. Parasitol. 1; 83.

Mathey, W.J. jr (1955) Malaria in canaries. Vet. Med, 50; 369-370.
        Schrag, L., Enz, H. Klette, H. and Messinger, H. (1985) Healthy Pigeons 5th Engl. rev. ed.; 66.

Stabler, R.M. (1948) Protection in pigeons against virulent Trichomonas gallinae acquired by infection with milder strains. J. Parasitol. 34;150.

Stabler, R.M. (1951) Effect of Trchomonas gallinae from diseased doves on clean domsetic pigeons. J. Parasitol. 37; 473.

Stabler, R.M. (1954) Trichomonas gallinae: A review. Exptl. Parasitol. 3; 368.

Stone, W.B. and Jones, D.E. (1969) Trichomoniasis in captive sparrow hawks. Bull. Wildlfe Disease Assoc. 5; 147.

Wallis, A.S (1991) Common conditions of domestic pigeons. In Practice May, 1991.
Whitney, L.F. (1969) Keep your pigeons flying. 2nd. ed.; 145, 138-139.

Chapter 7: Parasitic diseases.

Lapage, G. (1962) Monnig's Veterinary Helminthology and Entomology.
5th Edition, Balliere, Tindall and Cox, London.
Wehr, E.E. and Hwang, J.C. (1964) The life cycle and morphology of Ascaridia columbae (Gmelin, 1970) Travassos, 1913 (Nematoda: Ascaridiae) in the domestic pigeon (Columba livia domestica). J. Parasitol. 50:131

Chapter 8: Neoplasms.

DeVriese, L. (1986) Diergeneesk. Memorandum 33 no 1; 47.
Tudor, D.C. (1991) Pigeon Health and Disease. 1st Ed. 7:143-145.

Chapter 9: Toxins and poisons

Devriese, L. (1986) Diergeneesk. Memorandum 33 no 1:42.
Clarke, E.G.C. (1975) Poisoning in Veterinary Practice.
Association of the British Pharmaceutical Industry, London.
Joyce, R. (1970) Ontspan met wedvlugduiwe. 1ste druk 95-96.
Tafelberg Uitgewers, Kaapstad.

Garner, R.J. (1963) Veterinary Toxicology. 2nd Ed. 229-275, .
Stam, J.W.E. (1986) Personal communication.
Trainer, D.O. and Karstad, L. (1960) Salt poisoning in Wisconsin wildlife. J. Am. Vet. Med. Assoc. 136(1):14.
Vansalen, V. (1973) Vitamines en Dopings in de Duivensport. 1ste Druk. Uitgevery Ankh Hermes bv, Deventer.
Vogel, K. (1980) Die Taube – Biologie, Haltung, Futterung, Deutscher Landwirtschaftsverslag, Berlijn -DDR.

Chapter 10: Breeding problems

Devriese, L. (1986) Diergeneesk. Memorandum 33 no 1: 11.
Vermeijen, L and Aerts, J. (1969) Communique – Hoe wy ze keuren. 5de Druk. Jos Adriaenssens, p.v.b.a., Antwerpen. 12.

Chapter 11: Micellaneous diseases and conditions.

Axworthy, A.X. (1970) Pigeon Care and Protection.

Buttner, E.E. (1968) Arginine deficiency link with feather plucking. Cage & Aviary Birds 134:256.

Devriese, L. (1986) Diergeneesk. Memorandum 33 no 1: 10, 61-66.

Kendeigh, S.C (1962) Personal Communication to C.I. Tollefsen – Nutrition in Ed. M.L. Petrak Diseases of Cage and Aviary Birds. 2nd Ed. 7; 241-242.

Lemahieu, P. (1986) Personal communication.

Minsky, L. and Petrak, M.L. (1982) Metabolic and Miscellaneous Conditions. in Ed. M.L. Petrak Diseases of Cage and Aviary Birds. 2nd Ed. 28; 638-645.

Riddle, O., Hollander, W.F. and Schooley, J.P. (1945) A race of hermaphrodite-producing pigeons. Anat. Rec. 91: 401-423.

Whitney, L.F. (1969) The Basis of Breeding Racing Pigeons. 1st Ed. 99-100. Faber and Faber, London.

Chapter 18: Antimicrobials

Conradie, R.C. (1991) Commonly used Medications in Racing Pigeons. .A. Racing Pigeon/ Posduif Vol 2:6, 20-21.

Daykin, P.W. (1960) Veterinary Applied Pharmacology and Therapeutics. Bailliere, Tindall and Cox, London.

Devriese, L. (1986) Diergeneesk. Memorandum 33 no 1: 61-66.

Fris, C en Wagenaar-Schaafsma, A.E. (1981) Red. Compendium – Behandelingsadviezen voor ziekten bij nut- en sierpluimvee. 4de druk.

I.V.S. Index of Veterinary Specialities (1993) 31:2 (June – August)

Schrag, L., Enz, H. Klette, H. and Messinger, H. (1985) Healthy Pigeons 5th Engl. rev. ed.;

Swan, G.E. (1987) Veterinary Pharmacology 700 Notes, Antimicrobials. Dept. Parmacology and Toxicology, Onderstepoort.

Chapter 19: Parasiticides

Devriese, L. (1986) Diergeneesk. Memorandum 33 no 1: 25, 61-66.

I.V.S. Index of Veterinary Specialities, (1993) 31:2 (June – August).

Fris, C en Wagenaar-Schaafsma, A.E. (1981) Red. Compendium – Behandelingsadviezen voor ziekten bij nut- en sierpluimvee. 4de druk.

Chapter 21: Vitamins, Minerals and Amino Acids.

Ferrando, R. and workers (1971) Ann. Nutr. Alim. 25:241-245

Joyce, R. (1970) Ontspan met wedvlugduiwe. 1ste druk 95-96.
   Tafelberg Uitgewers, Kaapstad.

Leash, A.M. and workers (1971) Lab. Animal Sci. 21:86-90

Vansalen, V. (1973) Vitamines en Dopings in de Duivensport. 1ste
   Druk. Uitgevery Ankh Hermes bv, Deventer.

Index

tetrameres, 35, 52, 56, 59, 125, 128-131, 136, 271

ticks, 149

toes, 53, 74, 93, 159, 165-166, 180, 195-196, 217, 224, 236

tongue, 30, 46-48, 98, 111, 116, 127, 137

trachea, 22-23, 26, 28-30, 49, 54, 56, 60, 64, 85, 114, 126, 145, 159, 186, 225

trichomoniasis, 28, 33, 36, 39, 47-48, 55-56, 58, 66, 76, 80-81, 86, 109, 111, 114-116, 119, 121, 172, 186, 204, 266

vaccines, 69-71, 76, 96-97

virus, 47, 55, 58-59, 63-65, 69-75, 78, 80-83, 85, 89-90, 117-118, 144, 152-153, 201, 210, 233, 268, 278

vitamin, 27, 37, 39, 57, 76, 93, 96, 108, 118, 164, 166, 170-171, 176, 180-182, 184, 246, 252, 281-292, 294

vitamin deficiency, 93, 252

wing, 24, 45, 61, 66, 72, 74, 85, 92-93, 95, 143, 145, 154, 186, 197-198, 214, 217, 220-221, 224, 228, 235, 239-240

worms, 18, 21, 34-35, 37, 48, 52, 56-57, 86, 107, 125-127, 129-135, 137-138, 140-141, 269, 271-272

yeast, 171, 246, 281-282, 284-286, 288-290

yellow liver disease, 33, 37, 200

yolk, 154, 175, 178-179, 183, 185, 189-192, 241